Reweaving Our Social Fabric
A Muslim Conference for the 21st Century
Granada, Spain
June 2019

Reweaving Our Social Fabric

A Muslim Conference for the 21st Century

Granada, Spain

June 2019

DIWAN PRESS

Classical and Contemporary Books on Islam and Sufism

FOUNDED IN 1975

Copyright © Diwan Press Ltd., 2020 CE/1442 AH

Reweaving Our Social Fabric

Published by: Diwan Press Ltd.
                                311 Allerton Road
                                Bradford
                                BD15 7HA
                                UK
Website: www.diwanpress.com
E-mail: info@diwanpress.com

Authors: Ibtisaam Ahmed, Aisha Bewley, Rahima Brandt,
                                Khadija Martinez, Tahira Narbona, Rabea Redpath
Edited by: Khalila Grundl
Typeset by: Abdassamad Clarke
Cover design by: Khalila Grundl, Abdassamad Clarke
Cover Illustration by: Saida Nuria Aragoneses
Photographs by: Dr. Fatima Ahmed, Khalila Grundl, Atiqah Addy, Fatima Perez
                                and Selima Powell

A catalogue record of this book is available from the British Library.

ISBN-13:   978-1-908892-59-1 (paperback)
                                978-1-908892-99-7 (ePub and Kindle)

CONTENTS

ACKNOWLEDGEMENTS

This publication has been a collaborative project of many helpers whose efforts in transcribing, translating, editing and proofreading the talks, sharing ideas and inspiration regarding title and cover, has been immensely helpful and greatly appreciated.

Everything is everything
What is meant to be, will be
After winter, must come spring
Change, it comes eventually

Lauryn Hill 'Everything is Everything'

This booklet contains a series of talks that formed part of "Encounters for Change" that took place in June 2019 in Granada, Spain.

The scope of our conference was ambitious and the substance of these talks is of vital significance to all freethinking men and women. Since then, our situation has changed.

We are now all witness to an unfolding of events that is predictable, yet alarming. The themes of resilience, internet surveillance, health and autonomy, the increasing authoritarian nature of governments, social welfare, the removal of the Divine from society, economic devastation and civil unrest are no longer theoretical suppositions, but questions that require our reflection and action in ensuring our survival.

The modern world has been left no choice but to examine its myriad of unresolved contradictions. This plunge into chaos has awakened in many people the need to re-evaluate the structures we are complicit in upholding and the values upon which our lives are constructed. This means that conversations which were once deemed abstract and severed from the common sense realities of everyday life, are now vital in ensuring a way out of the toxic miasma of an age characterized by violence, social decay, nihilism and a disregard for the dignity of the human being.

This has made the publication of these talks absolutely crucial. Our hope is that this contribution is a means of beginning a dialogue around alternatives and creating a vision for a different future. The purpose of the publication is to share the analysis of our speakers – some of the contents presented will find resonance with the reader and others will not. Similarly, proposed solutions might also be different. But the goal has not been to achieve systematic uniformity; rather it is to begin a journey of questioning, self-reflection and commitment to action.

In this way, what we have done with the Encounters Conference is what the woman who is connected with the Divine has always done — she holds up a mirror of what she sees around her and provides counsel on how it can be changed. The Final Messenger ﷺ said, "The deen is nothing but good counsel." He ﷺ also said that if the end of the world should come upon you while you were planting a tree — continue to plant the tree.

IBTISAAM AHMED
CAPE TOWN, SOUTH AFRICA
JULY 2020

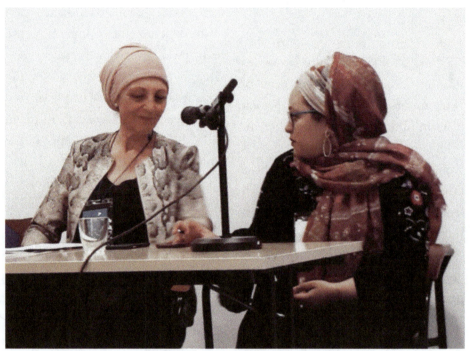

Khadija Martinez and Ibtisaam Ahmed

Welcome and Introduction

Firstly, I want to welcome everybody and thank you for the effort you have made to be here, especially those who have travelled from far away. It is an honour to have you all here, and it is such a pleasure that we can all come together. We have among us two non-Muslim guests, both professors of Anthropology and old friends of mine. We thought it would be beneficial for them to attend this conference, and for us to have them here with us.

The idea for this meeting arose at the last moussem in Cape Town, during a conversation in the kitchen among a large group of women as we prepared a women's breakfast. We ate in a beautiful place with views of the sea, and perhaps that is what inspired us.

Although the viewpoints during that discussion differed greatly, it was clear to us that there was a need to come together, talk about the issues and reach common positions.

I want to thank Ra'is Abu Bakr Rieger, who immediately supported and encouraged us when we presented him with the idea, and also Amir Umar of Granada who offered full access to the mosque when we came to him with the idea and has given us his unconditional support.

The main thing that I got from that initial discussion in Cape Town was that, as Muslim women, we are living in a socially complicated time, and it's very important for us to have a clear approach to be able to tackle the challenges of our time. We are going to have discussions after each talk, and, naturally, we will chat in the corridors and over lunch and so on — in other words, there will be plenty of exchange to get ideas flowing! Please note that we have women from all five continents here with us. It is a unique opportunity for us to create bonds with each other and hear different perspectives, which will benefit us all.

This conference is highly significant — not only for those who have worked hard to organise it but for all of us — and your presence here confirms that these are topics of interest. We need to establish positions which will help us to practice our deen correctly in the times we live in, and to best transmit it to a decadent society immersed in nihilism and in which so many are desperately seeking an alternative so that they can live in harmony.

GRANADA, SPAIN, JUNE 2019

I'd like to share with you an experience we had a few months ago. I and members of our community were invited to a conference on Islam, and this was attended by members of other Muslim communities. What surprised me the most was the unfortunate discourse into which the umma is falling – it is defensive, meaning that the kuffar are setting the terms of the debate. We cannot be apologetic. We cannot get trapped in a negative discourse in which we begin by saying "Islam is *not* this" or "We Muslims are *not* that".

I was also surprised by the prevalence of the term "Islamophobia". Wasn't Islamophobia really born as soon as the message of Islam was revealed? Because the first person to be attacked for being a Muslim was the Rasool ﷺ in Mekka. Even his own family attacked him. His people persecuted him to the point that he had to run away because they wanted to kill him. Isn't this Islamophobia?

The problem is when we Muslims assume that the narrative of the kuffar is real, because if we believe their assertion that they are democratic, open and tolerant, then we just end up running after them, asking them to fulfil those claims, and we forget that in the Qur'an it says the kuffar will not stop until they make us abandon our deen. In addition, the wars and the conflicts in so many Muslim countries are leading us to adopt a victim or beggar mentality, utterly contrary to the spirit of the deen!

During the conference in Seville, Nietzsche was quoted. He said that when we act as a reaction to what someone else does, we are acting as slaves. Only when a voice is born from a very clear intention and from a clear and positive will is it the action of a free being. With that in mind, I just wanted to remind us to be very aware of what we have. Not only has Allah gifted us with the deen, He has also given us clear guidance for the times we live in. Shaykh Abdalqadir has given us a clear methodology and tools. We are part of a community whose history encompasses half a century and four generations. We have achieved many things, on a personal level as well as with regard to our families and the social arena. We have also made a lot of mistakes; I hope that we have learned from them and that they will not be repeated in future generations.

> *We cannot get trapped in a negative discourse in which we begin by saying "Islam is not this" or "We Muslims are not that".*

Alhamdulillah wash-shukrulillah, many people are coming to the mosque. I've had the opportunity to meet many people from all around the world – when they come asking about the deen, I get called because I'm just around the corner! I would like to share with you another experience of mine. A lady who had come from a different continent contacted us, said the shahada and then stayed on to live with us for a time. One day, with tears in her eyes, she said to me, "Khadija, what you have is a reality, it is not theory. And the proof of this is the generations who have come after you and who are continuing the work. Please, please take this out to the world because there are so many people who are in dire need of what you have!" The ball is in our court, we have no option but to play it.

Please, let's play like women and bring out that femininity which is sorely missing in our world today.

I ask Allah that nobody leaves this encounter without having learned something new, and that each one of us has renewed energy and a firm commitment to implement what she has taken from these discussions. Amin!

KHADIJA MARTINEZ

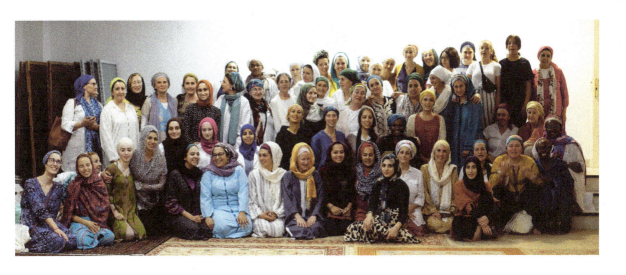

GRANADA, SPAIN, JUNE 2019

We could start this talk with a history of western powers colonialising Muslim regions and imposing Western values on them by force or by indoctrination and educating their upper class to emulate them as the English did, or through blatant force and exploitation in the case of other colonial powers, all of which would be historically interesting. There was the replacement of Shari'a with secular law, relegating religion to a private matter of secondary importance, and changing what is of primary importance in the course of exploitation of natural resources. There was a diminution of the position of women, reflecting the European attitudes at the time – particularly the Victorian English – and this has endured for a long time. All of this is true, but in the current situation focusing on the wrongs of the past results in blaming the situation in which we now find ourselves on the past and thinking that there should be reparations for these injustices. And this results in our ignoring, or at least passing over, the more pressing problems of the present.

> *The business facing us is, in fact, much more profound and more acute than memories of past injustices because the colonialists themselves have now been 'colonialised' by their own system.*

The business facing us is, in fact, much more profound and more acute than memories of past injustices because the colonialists themselves have now been 'colonialised' by their own system. The old adage of the 'Revolution devouring their own children' still holds true. This is not a conspiracy theory based on a sinister cabal plotting in a darkened room. It is simply based on what inevitably results from ruthlessly exploiting people to make money and this necessarily results in a small group of people being in control. It is market logic. Another group have replaced the older power nexus – as is the normal course of things. There was no plotting to make it so – it just resulted logically from a system fuelled by usury. It is the logic that stems from the acceptance of usury that provides the impetus in the current economic system.

The definition of colonialisation is: 'seeking to extend or retain authority over other peoples or territories, generally with the aim of opening trade opportunities.' By authority or control now I mean having the ability to influence and shape people's behaviour. Examples of this are sending you an ad when you are full of endorphins at the end of a run and therefore ready to click on 'buy', or putting a particular phrase into your Facebook news feed which acts as a trigger for you, or micro-targeting based on your Facebook profile.

There are several vectors of this colonialisation, the internet and education being the most evident of them. Education has already played its role in providing the moulded receptors ready for programming, and now social media is progressing with the process at a very rapid pace and reinforcing it. Perhaps even our neural patterning is being rewritten.

Things are now moving on in a manner that had not been planned or foreseen by anyone. We are now in a system which was initially called digital capitalism which now has moved into what is designated as 'surveillance capitalism'. Its function, as we said, is dictated by the logic of economic interests. It has been a process which has brought us to where we are by a series of decisions, all based, of course, on capitalist financial goals, which are based on

a system fuelled by exploitation. Shoshana Zuboff has written on this in *The Age of Surveillance Capitalism* if someone wants to read all the details.

It has been said that we are now living through the most profound transformation since Gutenberg's invention of printing in about 1439. What did that, at the time, a seemingly innocuous attempt to facilitate access to information, result in? The Reformation, the undermining of the power of the Catholic Church, the Enlightenment, the rise of modern science, the demise of the old order, new industries, and a profound change in how we view ourselves. We are now living through just such a time.

The shift to where we are now stems from the dot.com bust in 2001 where the prices of internet-based companies reached a peak and then crashed. Due to investor pressure, or panic, Google's leaders decided to stop being hostile to the idea of advertising, which they had been in the past. After that they decided to boost their ad revenue by applying Google's ability to analyze its cache of behavioural data to make ads relevant to users, and hence more valuable to advertisers. Before this decision, that information was basically considered to be waste material. A seemingly innocuous decision had far-reaching consequences. They increased their data capture, which had just been a by-product of little use, and used new methods to uncover even more personal data and infer more personal information from the existing data. This is then analysed for meaning in order to predict future behaviour. Lots of algorithms!

Zuboff refers to it as a 'behavioural futures market' and we ourselves are the raw materials for the market, which is free for them. She likens it to someone discovering virgin forest which no one owns and is ready for logging. Google entered into a new market realm which had no laws governing it, and their revenue in three years increased by 3,590 percent, from $86 million to $3,2 billion. This technique of information extraction moved from Google into Facebook when Sheryl Sandberg, a Google executive, became Zuckerberg's number two in Facebook in 2008. Amazon has followed the same course with their algorithms as I am sure we have all experienced after browsing their website, and now with Alexa. Everything 'smart' provides data to the providers. And it has moved on beyond the behemoths

Suffice it to say, that everything you do online or on your smart phone or with smart devices provides raw material which will be used to predict your future behaviour, and mould it. It makes old-time colonialisation look amateur.

of the internet. The little guys are doing it too, now.

What is the term for those who have grown up in the digital age? Digital natives. Older people who predate it are called digital immigrants. Back to echoes of the language used in colonialisation. In colonialisation, there is what is known as the 'conquest pattern', the first step of which is legalistic justification in the form of a declaration. And the surveillance capitalists have indeed declared our private transactions and experience to be theirs once they have been rendered into the form of data. They exploit us as a resource. You aren't even the consumers anymore, but the consumed. So far only the EU has put up any real barriers for them with GDPR, which is the General Data Protection Regulation.

Suffice it to say, that everything you do online or on your smart phone or with smart devices provides raw material which will be used to predict your future behaviour, and mould it. It makes old-time colonialisation look amateur. This is about controlling your autonomy, your behavior and even your thought processes. And you don't even notice it. As Zuboff quotes Mark Weiser, who said this back in 1999: 'The most profound technologies are those that disappear. They weave themselves into the fabric of everyday life until they are indistinguishable from it.' Everything is now raw data: your facial expressions, your use of exclamation marks, how you say something. And you don't notice it at all. To quote Zuboff:

> In order to achieve these economies of action, machine processes are configured to intervene in the state of play in the real world among real people and things.

These interventions are designed to augment prediction products in order that they approximate certainty by "tuning," "herding," and conditioning the behaviour of individuals, groups, and populations. These economies of action apply techniques that are as varied as inserting a specific phrase into your Facebook news feed, timing the appearance of a BUY button on your phone with the rise of your endorphins at the end of a run, shutting down your car engine when an insurance payment is late, or employing population-scale behavioral micro-targeting drawn from Facebook profiles (*as in elections*). Indeed, the notorious manipulations of the data firm Cambridge Analytica, which scandalized the world in 2018, simply appropriated the means and methods that are now both standard and necessary operations in the surveillance capitalism arsenal.

You can change your privacy settings and get rid of Alexa, or Siri or Google Assistant and turn off your tracking via Bluetooth, but that is not really the point. It has really gone beyond that. Of course, even if your GPS is turned off, smartphones are using local Wi-Fi networks which can locate you, and even if the Wi-Fi is also turned off, the phone, with its functions within the operating system, can be used to triangulate your cell signal to roughly locate you.

But nonetheless technology is a tool – a very sophisticated tool, but a tool nevertheless. And Google and then Amazon and Facebook did not come up with this exploitation on their own. The clue is in the second part of the name – capitalism, which is built on usury and chance. It developed from the logic of a system based on usury.

And lest we simply attribute this to a totalitarian Big Brother, she says:

> 'There is no brother here of any kind, big or little, evil or good—no family ties, however

grim. Instead this new global apparatus is better understood as a *Big Other* that encodes the "otherized" viewpoint of radical behaviorism as a pervasive presence (*it is everywhere, but it's not an individual*).

"Instrumentalization" denotes the social relations that orient the puppet masters to human experience, as surveillance capital overrides the long- standing reciprocities of market democracy, wielding its machines to transform us into the raw material for its own production.

It's not a conspiracy – it's just market logic. It affects the entire system.

So why is this tailoring things to your personal preferences so terrible even though it is clearly very creepy? It is because what they get is never enough and now they want to modify behavior to achieve their desired commercial outcomes. What is the point of all this information unless they can profit from it?

So the goal is now behavior modification. It is not about compelling conformity with social norms, although that does happen with social media, but to produce behaviour that reliably leads to predicted commer-

> *The clue is in the second part of the name — capitalism, which is built on usury and chance. It developed from the logic of a system based on usury.*

cial results. The research director of Gartner, a business advisory firm, said that 'the internet of things' – such as your refrigerator and all the other appliances in your house – will serve as 'a key enabler in the transformation of business models from 'guaranteed levels of performance' to 'guaranteed outcomes'.

This started with Facebook's emotional contagion experiment in 2012 where the newsfeed was manipulated for a week, some people receiving mostly happy or positive words, and some receiving sadder input, and then what they themselves posted was checked. Basically they wanted to see if they could make you feel bad without you noticing – and they did. There have been other experiments like self-censorship, effects of sharing, the role of social networks in information diffusion, and of course their role in the elections. Pokeman Go was also such a test of influencing behaviour: they could get you to go wherever they wanted you to go. The goal of this is to automate us and find out the optimum way of doing so.

Perhaps the Dajjal is represented by this process. Allahu a'lam. If so, hadith tells us that protection from the Dajjal is found in reciting the first ten or last ten ayahs of *Surat al-Kahf*. The first ten tell us about the importance of the revelation and end with the beginning of the story of the People of the Cave who sought refuge in Allah and in the cave. To which I will return.

The pervasiveness of this technology is, of course, alarming. Perhaps the reaction is to throw away your smart phone and run screaming for the hills. But you're still trackable and findable – satellite, drones, thermal sensors and so forth. You will be found eventually. The answer isn't out there. It is inside us.

If we read the beginning of the *Way of Muhammad* – and remember how long ago Shaykh Abdalqadir wrote this book, fifty years ago:

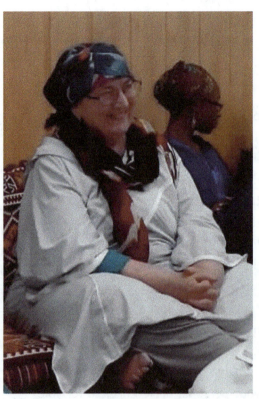

Aisha Bewley

whatever particular individuality you may imagine you have over and against those millions of others. You have an idea of how

> 'There is only one method by which you can approach the sufic sciences and that is to start, tabula rasa, by putting away the whole world-picture and value structure which has formed you until now and which is completely the result of your social and historical imprinting which you share with millions of others,

things are, and how you are, how things should be and how you should be. Interposed between you and reality is a functioning fluctuating conceptualization of existence that, mingled with your personal emotional responses to event and personality, make up what you think is both 'you' and 'your world'.

Which is describing exactly what happens to our view of ourselves now.

As we have said, this view of yourself, which is illusionary, is now being deliberately manipulated by the 'Big Other'. There needs to be a true realisation of tawhid, reflection, and the construction of good character and action. The extent of the programming I have mentioned makes a lot of the traditional approaches of no real consequence. 'Education' as a social process, and by this I mean formal education, has been already co-opted by the process. We need to go deeper. Dhikr is required as an inoculation against what is happening all around us.

In some ways, as Muslims we have to be even more aware because of the false sense of security that we are safe because we have the *shahadah*, but the reality of that *shahadah* depends on whether it is just with our finger and on our tongues without being firmly rooted in our hearts and lodged in our consciousness. It requires a deep and profound understanding of tawhid in the heart that manifests in behavior on both a micro and macro level.

So the question is what to do? What am I here for? Having named the problem, there are two strands we must hold onto. The first is tawhid which must be at a more profound level in your being and constantly reinforced because the Big Other is constantly after you as well. Shaykh Abdalqadir, in a talk on futuwwa, says:

> *The fuqara must ask always to be in change. The du'a of the Sufis is, "O Allah, keep me in change."*

> The fuqara must ask always to be in change. The du'a of the Sufis is, "O Allah, keep me in change." Keep me always changing because everything is changing and every day Allah is on a new creation. You must be renewing and renewing yourself. You have to always be in change. You must remember that the company of the fuqara is the highest company. You must keep each other company. You must

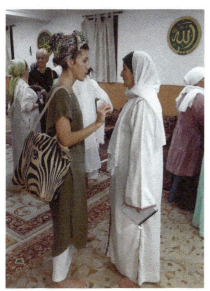

Rabea Redpath, right, in conversation with an attendee at the conference travel to other places where there are fuqara. You must sit with the fuqara in every place. You must be an example to them and take example from them when you meet people of quality. Seek the people of knowledge, seek the people of love of Allah, subhanahu wa ta'ala, and the people of love of Rasul ﷺ. To take the adab of the great ones you have to sit with them, you have to sit with the people of knowledge. It is by your company that you are purified. Tasawwuf is keeping company, then tasawwuf is listening, then tasawwuf is acting upon what you hear. There is only one enemy and that is your self. The nafs has nothing good in it. The worst of all things to the Sufis is the recognition of their own good qualities over and against that of other people – it is what sets them back and smashes them on the rocks of destiny. You must not look at your good qualities.

You must consider them something that in themselves have been spoiled even by your being conscious of them. You do not look at your self.

Now this is for you personally, but this is not enough. We need to then move out to the macro- dimension or, if you like, the political dimension.

The tenth ayah of *Surat al-Kahf* is: '*When the young men took refuge in the cave and said, 'Our Lord, give us mercy directly from you and open the way for us*

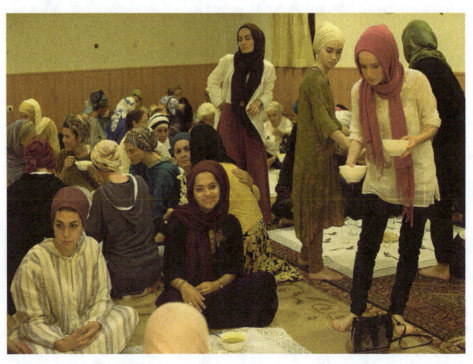

to right guidance in our situation.' This is seeking to apply tawhid in one's current situation, and they were in such a dire situation that their only recourse was to seek refuge in the cave. This is the source of the term *futuwwa*. Sometimes translated as noble chivalry, it comes from *fitya*, the plural of *fata*, young man, as referred to in this ayah. *Futuwwa* is what happens when the human being is transformed by tawhid. These young men asked for guidance, for illumination from Allah, after they had gathered together in the cave, which was cutting themselves off from idolatry. This Cave is what Shaykh Abdalqadir, taking the term from Ernst Jünger, calls the Waldgang, the forest, the non-temporal: this is going into tawhid. The person who does this is the Waldgänger (Forester) or the new Bedouin. These terms are all representations of this idea of the individual finding his or her identity in relation to this world, and that entails finding his or her relationship to the Divine, to Allah, in a profound transformative way. After this transformation, the human being becomes a transformative force himself because

> *Any impulse to unify is taught to be socially disruptive. The only group activities permitted are groups of common interest in sexual practices, sports and concerts.*

the sum is greater than the parts.

This then moves to a larger group, just as the young men in the Cave were a group. Or in the other instances in the Qur'an where the term is used, Ibrahim took his family and relatives on Hijra, and in the case of Musa, he took the tribe of Israel. The process moves from the individual to a larger group, applying what has been learned in the Cave. This has been discussed by Shaykh Abdalqadir. In referring to 'Asabiyya, the sense of 'tribal' unity mentioned by Ibn Khaldun, Shakyh Abdalqadir says:

'It has in it also a moral evaluation as in the term 'Futuwwa', chivalry or nobility of character. Asabiyya unites men to find the power to act and transform and command. If its motor power is high its brotherhood is raised higher. If the binding factor (*religio* – to bind together) is there, that is Divine religion, it is, that being its highest possibility, assured a triumph.'

He also says:

Without Asabiyya the Bedouin remain isolated individuals. The slave is alone. His religion, he has been programmed to accept, is his own private privilege –

nobody else's business. This guarantees that they will not pose a threat, except as isolated individuals, that is, criminals.

The Bedouin who cannot engender Asabiyya among themselves are assured continual slavery. Any impulse to unify is taught to be socially disruptive. The only group activities permitted are groups of common interest in sexual practices, sports and concerts.

So the secret in *Kahf* is pointed out. Once fully immersed in tawhid, one must join forces with a larger group to see tawhid implemented in the wider community. This would entail amirs, zakat collection and distribution, etc. This is an ongoing process because we do not have it. Shaykh Abdalqadir has been encouraging it, indeed rather forcefully encouraging it, but it is a work in progress, and it is one that we must not forget or neglect.

And I will end with a quote from *The Entire City*, by Shaykh Abdalqadir:

'The inner circle of human society is not the law of the land, but it does not overthrow the law. Society has its structures and needs its leaders, and as we have established they may at one point raise up a leader and at another, a ruling group and at another, the

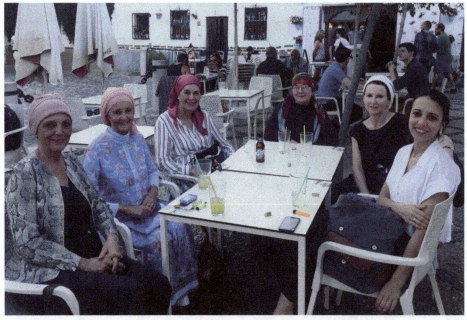

From left to right: Khadija Martinez, Rabea Redpath, Zulaikha Lund, Aisha Bewley, Rahima Brandt, and Aisha Hernandez.

forms may collapse. However, the governance of society where it is the responsibility of a man (or a woman) in his time, at the same time a man must live to the best of his knowledge. The lived life is dependent on the company of a few. Divine Messengers confirmed or revised societal law but they drew their strength from a chosen circle of quality. Jesus's followers were gathered at a divinely given table to feast their brotherhood. The final Messenger names ten men as assured the Garden in the Unseen, they were the chosen and the best of men.'

So what it is pointing out is that you go from yourself to a smaller group, and then you try to spread it out wider among society.

AISHA BEWLEY

Resilience in a Changing Landscape
Women in the 21st Century

I would like to begin my talk by reading out part of a poem written in 1973 by an African-American Muslim woman named Sonia Sanchez. The poem is a declaration on Muslim womanhood as it intertwines freedom with spirituality which is fitting for many of the themes I will be discussing today. It is called *We Are Muslim Women*.

WE ARE MUSLIM WOMEN
wearing garments of the righteous
recipients of eternal wisdom
followers of a Divine man and Message
listen to us
as we move thru the eye of time
rustling with loveliness
listen to our wisdom
as we talk in the Temple of our Souls.

WE ARE MUSLIM WOMEN
dwellers in light
new women created from the limbs of Allah
We are the shining ones
coming from dark ruins
created from the eye of Allah:
And we speak only what we know
And we do not curse God
And we keep our minds open to light
And we do not curse God
And we chant Alhamdulilah

And we do not curse God
WE ARE MUSLIM WOMEN

I have made the choice to discuss resilience instead of resistance, rebellion or revolution – and by the end of the talk I hope my reasons for doing so will become clear. The word 'resilience' is derived from the Latin word meaning to 'recoil or rebound', *re* meaning 'back', and *salire* meaning 'to jump or leap'. We understand resilience in a figurative sense, but in the 19th century, 'resilience' was a technical term used by watchmakers to denote the flexible qualities of internal components that prevented excessive vibration. By the 1850s, 'resilient' was used to describe being resistant or not susceptible to something. It has also meant elasticity. Today we associate resilience with survival, strength and the ability to withstand difficulties.

Resilience can be understood in two ways:

- preparation or organization in anticipation of an oncoming crisis
- recovery or reconstruction after a defeat or a crisis

When examining the situation in which we find ourselves, it has become clear that resilience for the woman today encompasses both of these things. On the one hand we are trying to come out of the ruins of ideas on women's liberation that have failed us, and at the same time we are preparing for what is coming in order to ensure our survival.

As women of the 21st century, we must be aware of our history and how we got here. There is a particular narrative of women that has dominated modern thought originating in the Western world, but eventually finding traction the world over. So at the outset I must emphasize the gift that among us at this conference we have women who grew up and knew life before the 'Women's Movement' of the 1960s; women who were at the forefront of feminism; women who grew up enjoying the fruits of equal opportunity; and women who have come of age in the era of #metoo and a feminism which emphasizes intersectionality and the view that one's biology is not determinative of gender. It means that we have a true spectrum of views and perceptions and this is im-

> *On the one hand we are trying to come out of the ruins of ideas on women's liberation that have failed us and at the same time we are preparing for what is coming in order to ensure our survival.*

portant, because it protects us from dismissing certain experiences out of hand, without a broader, contextual understanding.

I don't think that any of these movements are valueless and there are certainly lessons from which we may take, even though feminism is sometimes seen as passé or irrelevant or quite frankly, uninteresting. It is clear that there is a lot of confusion around this topic. On the one hand, women are told: you don't need any of this because Islam guarantees you your rights. This is frustrating because these rights are

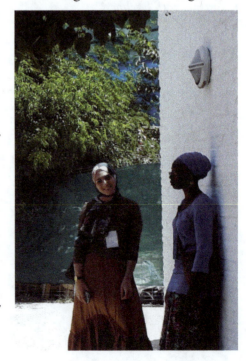

not always enacted and upheld. On the other hand, we see an increase in people trying to reduce Islam to a feminist project via selective readings and interpretations of the Qur'an and hadith.

Simone de Beauvoir in the introduction to *The Second Sex* written in 1949, says the following:

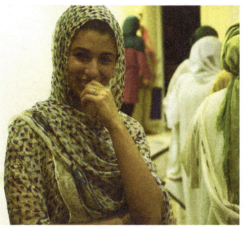

"I hesitated a long time before writing a book on women. The subject is irritating, especially for women; and it is not new. Enough ink has flowed over the quarrel about feminism; it is almost over; let's not talk about it anymore. Yet it is still being talked about."

Writing 70 years ago, what could Simone de Beauvoir have meant when she said that she believed that the quarrel about feminism was almost over? De Beauvoir was in fact referring to first-wave feminism or the suffragette movement. Outwardly, the movement was about women gaining the right to vote, but at a deeper level it was a challenge that women presented to the world: they could be in the public sphere, they could in fact move and negotiate the world. Yet many of these early feminists greatly admired men and did not feel the need to deride the great contributions of men to philosophy, politics and art. Instead they saw an opportunity to demonstrate what they were capable of bringing to society if certain barriers are removed. It is also crucial to note that these women did not, by any means, play the role of the victim. Theirs was a fight for a certain measure of autonomy, equal opportunity and breathing space in the shadow of Victorian bourgeois sensibilities. To take a lesson from these early first-wave feminists, I quote Sarah Grimké, an American suffragette who said, *"I ask no favour for my sex, all I ask of our brethren is that they take their feet off our necks!"*

The outbreak of World War I resulted in the decline of the women's movement as a political project, but the visibility of women certainly continued into the 1920s and 1930s, particularly seen in the work of witty writers and emerging starlets of the screen who reveled in jazz and dance. The short boyish hairstyles were matched with dark lipstick and a smoldering gaze – a woman at once emancipated yet simultaneously still a creature of mystery.

Much of this visibility of women had to do with the cataclysmic sense of disillusion felt after the horrors of WWI because it created an 'anti-authority sentiment', which weakened the status of the father-figure found in government, religion and the nuclear family. But the emergence of a powerful and accomplished woman was halted by the Great Depression in the United States and the rise of fascism in Europe. World War II made it a necessity for women to work while men were fighting at the front. The end of the war meant that women were expected to step aside. This, of course was an injustice done to women, but we also cannot ignore the reality that there was a deep need and longing for society to return to the comfort of domesticity after the trauma of two World Wars. The family was once again placed center stage, but the suffocating atmosphere of the 1950s bred discontent amongst women – giving rise to second wave feminism.

> *For many women living outside Europe and North America, feminism seemed to be a mere extension of an imperial and colonial legacy in which indigenous practices and beliefs were once more seen as repugnant and archaic.*

Second wave feminism is the kind of feminism we are most familiar with – it was seen as a project of liberation that went alongside the movement for civil rights. Accessible contraception, legalized abortion and equal employment opportunities set the agenda. Betty Friedan and her bevy of dis-contented house-wives clashed with the younger more radical fem-inists who were predominantly left-wing and anti-war. But feminism was made less threatening and more reasonable by the likes of Gloria Steinem with her soothing voice, fashion sense and approachability. The great success of this movement was its concept of 'consciousness raising' both at the outward and inward dimensions. Gloria Steinem, reflecting on the need for women to turn inward wrote "We recognized what we ourselves had experienced, felt trust because of that truth and then were taken one step further."

The problem however, was that most second wave feminists remained looking only at the outer, dismissing what Sonia Sanchez called "the Temple of our Souls". The other fatal mistake was the

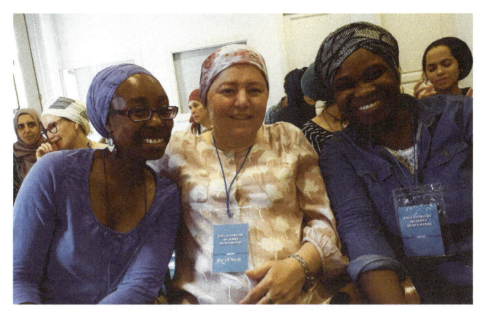

view and attitude towards men — instead of being time and place specific, second wave feminism chose to follow the route in which all men, everywhere throughout history were condemned. What we now might refer to today as #menaretrash.

The history I have thus far recounted has mostly centered on white women in the Western world, this has been deliberate as much of this movement was exactly that. For many women living outside Europe and North America, feminism seemed to be a mere extension of an imperial and colonial legacy in which indigenous practices and beliefs were once more seen as repugnant and archaic. The sisterhood, it appeared was only accessible to those women who played by the rules.

But in the 1980s, new players entered onto the scene. Feminism began to be tied into ideas emerging out of postcolonial studies and the study of racism. The climate was Edward Said's *Orientalism* and the big question asked by Gayatri Spivak in her influential article was "Can the subaltern speak?" Spivak posited that knowledge was exported to the Third world for financial gain and that research done on women who are "othered" is done entirely on colonial terms.

Another significant development was made by Kimberlé Crenshaw who introduced the term 'intersectionality', a term that looks at how race, class and sexual orientation overlap with gender. Unfortunately today, we now find ourselves caught in a myopic web of identity politics and a claim for victimhood. A contemporary self-described "dissident feminist", Jessa Crispin explains why and says, *"There are advantages to being labeled the victim. You are listened to, paid attention to. Sympathy is bestowed upon you."*

It is thus clear that the true liberation of women has yet to take place. Far from gaining political power, we have been robbed of it and we must acknowledge the catastrophe that has been made via rhetoric. While the experiences today of women the world over are depicted as a series of battles against a hegemony of globalization, capitalism and misogyny – the reality of what this means has been distorted. Depending on your geographic location, the politics of your country, your community or indeed your family – you may be experiencing a different struggle and this is why abstract ideas on women and freedom coming from universities often make no sense when looking at the real world and real people.

The discourse both in the academe and on social media is based on rhetoric and convoluted ideas on gender and sex that speak very little

> *The political woman, as we know, has shed her womanhood and has built up resentment towards men, while the pretty woman is free to do as she pleases, using her sexuality to find her value and move through the world.*

truth to the reality of women. I will describe a phenomenon that illustrates the point clearly:

At the Ivy League, those elite universities in the United States, one finds an immense discourse on social constructivism and gender. Men are censored into having no opinion and they dare not disagree with their female classmates. Anyone who does not toe the line of 'wokeness' is spoken down to. Women speak in a voice that is cold and cruel – reminiscent of Hillary Clinton in her failed bid for the American presidency in 2016. It is a voice that is snobby, condescending and void of any spontaneity. These young women at the elite universities are enabled by their wealth to disrespect potential detractors and enabled by their gender to have the final say on what is politically correct.

But when classes end on a Friday afternoon, something happens. The boys of the fraternities host parties at their frat houses and they travel around in packs – on the hunt. The apparently gutsy women melt into a puddle at the fraternity door once it is opened by a shirtless young man whose body is full of testosterone and alcohol. These men are allowed to behave like animals with their degrading rituals and view of women as disposable. When I asked a young woman why she participated in all this she said, "If I don't, I won't stand a chance with any of them".

From this example we see the inward split that is taking place within the modern woman:

the political woman
the pretty woman

In the classroom, there is a woman who is the 'pseudo man', but at the frat party there is the pretty woman, happy to be used and completely acquiescent to men. The political woman, as we know, has shed her womanhood and has built up resentment towards men, while the pretty woman is free to do as she pleases, using her sexuality to find her value and move through the world. It is true that beauty has and always will be a force in society playing an immense role in the nature and interaction of the relationship between men and women, but it is not beauty that I am referring to here.

The play, *The Face of Love* written in the 1950s, is a re-telling of the saga of Troy and is set post-WWII. We are all familiar with this myth and in particular the role of Helen of Troy – the face that launched a thousand ships and the war that ensues. The author brilliantly exposes what happens to Helen of Troy after 10 years.

Far from eternal youth and beauty, Helen is a decrepit woman, bitter and poisonous. Her beauty has faded and she comes to the profound realization that men have used her. Her worth was based on utility by men and it has left her with nothing.

Towards the end of the play she delivers a speech and the stage directions describe her as drunk "*her nightdress torn at the front. She is a harridan, ugly and glutted of her beauty, her eye make-up is heavy and her lipstick smudged. The crowd are amazed and frightened.*"

And then she delivers the following lines:

"*Now I will speak. Helen of Troy will talk and tell her story. I have been silent these ten years – now I will speak.*

Now Troy I'll tell you –

For ten years I have been prisoner in that Tower. Prisoner of Troy. My beauty and my youth held captive there. On a summer day ten years ago I lost my freedom – I have been prisoner ever since. And these ten years you've fought — fought for my freedom; well if freedom is a tower with high windows overlooking the sea — if freedom is being without friends and without the autumn countryside and the autumn beeches, if freedom is lusting with strange men and drinking into the night then you have not fought in vain because Helen has been free. For ten long years of hell I have been free..."

It is very clear that the state of this woman and her fate is absolutely brutal. The writer of this play was a 22-year-old Scotsman named Ian Dallas.

I raise all this because I am concerned about the way we currently perceive Muslim women in the public sphere. One of the advantages of social media is the relative ease with which anyone can tell their own story. Added to this is the overwhelming "representation" of Muslim women in mainstream media. But who are these women and what stories are they telling? We have reduced our visibility to an exercise in vanity. The voice of the modern Muslim woman is a "hijabi" — that awful word! — who has perfect eyebrows, glowing skin

> *Today's "modest Influencer" is simply "Helen in Hijab" because she is allowing herself to be used by forces of consumerism and capitalism.*

and an endorsement from companies whose labour practices and ethics are questionable at best and inhumane at worst. Today's "modest influencer" is simply "Helen in Hijab" because she is allowing herself to be used by forces of consumerism and capitalism. And once the allure fades – what will then be left of her?

This is what rhetoric has done, it has come up with slogans, hashtags and "movements" but has very little or no substance. The results are disastrous because women have been treated so appallingly and they have allowed men to do so. The theories dreamed up by those at the helm of "Womens' Studies" have demanded equality and have not demanded that women be honoured. There are very few places today where the woman is honoured. This word has itself been erased from our language because of its association with the evil attacks on women in places that have abandoned their Islam in order to practice their culture. These cultural practices can only be described as *jahiliyya*.

We must however, remember that rhetoric can succeed only in rhetorical terms. It is helpless against the archetype. It is helpless against nature.

Shaykh Abdalqadir as-Sufi writes something devastating in *The Time of the Bedouin*: *"Rhetoric, that terrible male weapon, was to silence once and for all that unlicensed gaiety and delight and pleasure that was womanhood."*

But we have chained ourselves to rhetoric of various kinds, of ideology of various kinds because this is what is demanded of us. Everywhere you turn you are told you must have an opinion, an ideology and it must be all-encompassing. You must take it all or leave it all. There is very little room in modern thought for *furqan* – discernment or discrimination. You are seen as quite unserious if you choose to take a bit from here and a bit from there. It is seen as a terrible weakness if you take the good from various people, ideas, culture and thought. This enslavement to rhetoric also means that one is unable to make a mistake. We have a "cancel culture" – you say one thing that is wrong or unfashionable and you are burnt at the stake for it. Twitter and other online platforms are frightening for this very reason.

Sidi Hakim Archuletta said something extraordinary, when talking about the body. He said "Flexibility increases resilience". So we have to have flexibility in finding solutions and forging a path forward for ourselves. We are of course deeply rooted in our *deen* and the Divine framework it provides, but we have to allow ourselves to engage in trial and error and to explore various options. It is flexibility which allows for this delight and pleasure that is womanhood.

In describing rhetoric as a male weapon, we are also being alerted to something in our own nature – rhetoric and sloganism is not part of woman's nature. We move by experience, we move by that which moves within us. As the Sanchez poem says, *"We speak only what we know"*.

Much of what we know is a direct result of the biology of femaleness, now more than ever, women must become more familiar with their own biology. Camille Paglia writes that "*Nature's cycles are women's cycles. Biological femaleness is a sequence of circular returns, beginning and ending at the same point.*" Nature's cycles and the woman's delicate proximity to both life and death in the process of childbirth speaks to this enormous knowledge. We move and are moved by that which we know to be true — so we can leave the slogans behind!

The situation I have described above calls for resilience after defeat. Shaykh Abdalqadir says in *The Interim is Mine* that it is fitting that "*where everything named actually stands for its opposite, the women's movement should be the mechanism for robbing women of their political power.*"

So we must emerge from this failure to become free women and recover true freedom. As Sonia Sanchez says "*We are the shining ones/ coming from dark ruins*".

The second aspect of resilience, however, is also necessary — we need to be prepared in anticipation of the coming crisis. Typically it is the nascent resilience, that provides the way out of the crisis. We have, in a few short years seen an exponential rise in nationalism and both extreme right and left wing politics, we are currently witnessing many civil wars and intrusions on the sovereignty of states. We are living in an environmental catastrophe and ours is an age of all kinds of extremes.

It is imminently clear then that the task is survival. Can we do it alone? No.

And here I look to our primordial origins, our earliest and first test as humanity and pointed out by one of my mentors, philosopher and law professor, Dr. Azizah al-Hibri.

The story of Adam and Eve: In the Judeao-Christian tradition, it was Eve who tempted Adam into disobeying God and so the founding myth is one where woman is seen as the crucial element in the downfall of man. This essentially sets up everything that follows in the Judeo-Christian tradition.

However, as Muslims, our understanding is that both were to blame equally. When Nabi Adam alayhi salam turned to Allah in tawba, the Quran tells us that he said "Rather we wronged ourselves". There is not any blame put onto woman. None at all.

Thus, for the Muslim, all of this is not about man and woman — it is

> *There is very little room in modern thought for furqan — discernment or discrimination (...) It is seen as a terrible weakness if you take the good from various people, ideas, culture and thought.*

about the human condition as a whole. And when confronted with a test, a challenge or indeed a crisis it has to be the case that we confront it together as free men and free women.

But what is the essence of a free woman? Shaykh Abdalqdir writes in *The Interim is Mine*, "The genuine power of woman, for good or evil, lies in her very persona."

What is our very persona? When reflecting on this or discussing it, we usually fall back into this concept of "authenticity" which is a nice enough word, but almost means nothing. What does it mean to be authentic?

> *To survive we have to come together and refine each other and bring out the qualities we see in each other. We must have roots that deep and unshakeable, but our branches must be flexible and able to move and adapt to changing conditions.*

I dare not assume to have the answer, but where abstract and intellectual reasoning may render confusion — when we turn to the seerah, there is always clarity. And every single Muslim has access to the seerah, Allah ta'ala has granted us this gift. We have all met people who have an understanding of even a handful of events that took place in the lifetime of the Prophet ﷺ which enables them to understand existence for what it truly is.

While reflecting on this, I was reminded of the great sahaba Khalid bin Walid. He was a military man and a

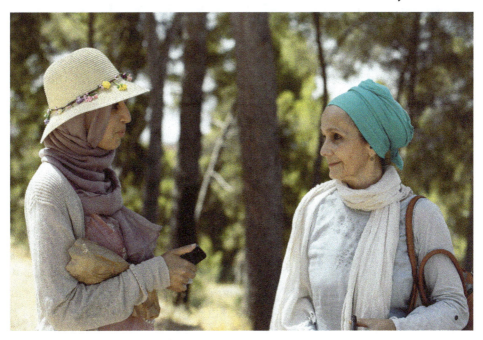

chief strategist at the Battle of Uhud. This battle was a devastating loss for the Muslims. The Prophet himself was injured, his uncle was killed as were many others of the sahaba. In fact, Uhud is something that we refer to very often, every time we sing the qasida *Nahnu Fi*. Shaykh Muhammad ibn al-Habib asks for a visit to every shaheed of Uhud and to the uncle of the Prophet.

So who was instrumental in defeating the Muslims at Uhud? Khalid bin Walid, he was a leader of the Meccans and it was his strategy that proved decisive. But then some time later – his heart is opened. He and two other men go to the Prophet and take their shahada. It is reported that he then asked the Prophet to ask Allah to forgive him. The Prophet tells Khalid that all his prior wrong actions have been forgiven. But Khalid insists and we know that the practice of our Prophet was that he never denied requests from people.

Allegedly, Khalid bin Walid also wanted to hand over his sword. Now, it must be understood that not only is Khalid's sword soaked in the blood of sahaba, it is also soaked in his trauma. He has killed the people from the group he is now a part of. It is a very heavy thing. Therefore one can understand why he would want to disassociate from that sword entirely. But as we all know, that is not what happened.

The following authentic hadith is found in Tirmidhi as mentioned by Ibn Hajar on the authority of Abu Huraira:

> "We descended with the Prophet ﷺ at a place, and people (companions) started passing by and the Prophet asked "Who is this?" and I said "It is so and so" until we reached Khalid. And the Prophet asked "Who is this?" and I replied "Khalid bin Walid" and the Prophet said, "What a great slave of Allah! This is a sword from the sword of Allah."

In other words, this man who had played a role in the death of the Prophet's uncle and so many sahaba became the Sayf Allah because the Prophet did not allow him to forget who he was. The Prophet never told him to give up the qualities he had, instead he was instructed to make use of them. He could not have been like Abu Bakr or Ali, it was not who he was. Khalid bin Walid was a brilliant soldier and strategist, Allah had created him that way, and the Prophet always validated his companions. It isn't about puffing up someone's ego, but he ﷺ recognized what people had and who they were.

In order to cultivate true resilience we must recognize what we have. Allah has created all of us with various capabilities and potentialities and when you activate these attributes of yourself and align them with what you know to be true – this is authenticity.

If you are not firmly rooted in who you are, any small wind or knock will leave you feeling defeated. A daffodil that is pretending to be a daisy will not be able to withstand the harsh elements of nature. To survive we have to come together and refine each other and bring out the qualities we see in each other. We must have roots that are deep and unshakeable, but our branches must be flexible and able to move and adapt to changing conditions.

We must also remember that our situation is by Allah, we rely on Him and we trust Him and we know that He is the author of our affair. We know that He is the One who makes us resilient and we do not curse our situation or the time we are living in.

As Sonia Sanchez so beautifully reminds us:

"And we do not curse God
And we chant Alhamdulilah
And we do not curse God
We are Muslim women."

IBTISAAM AHMED

Feminine Well-being in the Different Stages of Life: the Importance of the Tribe

Introduction

Everything that pertains to the health of women and their biological processes, such as menstruation, pregnancy, child-birth, breastfeeding and menopause, tend to be medicalised and treated as if they are illnesses.

There is a tendency to view women as unchanging, on a linear trajectory, unaffected by our cyclical processes that cause physical and emotional changes in us.

So, we take medication for period pain, epidurals for childbirth, anti-anxiety drugs for postnatal depression, anti-inflammatories for premenstrual syndrome (PMS), hormone replacement therapy for the menopause, and countless other drugs to avoid feeling the inevitable hormonal changes that take place throughout our lives.

Our instinctive needs that we have been given during these times, such as wanting to rest or withdraw during our periods, or the desire to not be separated from our newborn baby, are repressed and supplanted as we struggle to become Superwomen, a false and unattainable status that makes us anxious and fearful of not fulfilling expectations, not being accepted, not being productive, not being good enough, or of getting old or fat, and so on. Thus, we end up vulnerable victims of a system, in which the only comfort is consumerism.

To prevent this, we need the company of women with whom we share the same paradigm and a more complete view of existence.

When we share experiences with women of another generation who have already been there, they transmit their wisdom to us. We form a group, and the sense of belonging to a group produces endorphins. We are all enriched by this intergenerational connection, also because young women contribute up-to-date knowledge from universities and about new technologies.

All this will conduce to making us better people, and if we are mothers, it will help us with the responsibility of raising future adults who are healthier in every respect.

We also need to really know ourselves and understand how we function, the reasons for the things that we feel and experience, so that we can freely decide how to act and take an active attitude towards life.

GRANADA, SPAIN, JUNE 2019

We must keep in mind that we are biopsychosocial beings, a cohesion of body and mind interrelated by the nervous system and hormones.

Our being continuously reflects this unity: our thoughts and emotions influence the body through stress and somatisation (i.e. the manifestation of worries as physical symptoms); and conversely, when a part of the body is sick, it lets the brain know via the nervous system and alters the person's mood and can provoke emotions such as anger or sadness. This is why it is pointless to go on a pilgrimage from specialist to specialist looking at just one small part of the body to try to understand what is happening to us.

> *We must keep in mind that we are biopsychosocial beings, a cohesion of body and mind interrelated by the nervous system and hormones.*

We have to take an active approach to our health and healing, with Allah's permission.

For this purpose, we first of all need to understand how our body works, so that we can consciously embark on the journey through the different stages we experience during our lives.

The same things that happen to other women happen to us, but we deal with them from the perspective of our paradigm, as Muslim women of *fitra*, trusting in Allah and accepting our decree. This is true submission to our Lord.

Let's begin with a look at the various stages of our lives.

Menarche (first period)

When a girl gets her first period, her mother's attitude is crucial. If the mother has a healthy relationship with her body and explains menstruation as something natural, her daughter will not see the bleeding as something disgusting. Instead, she will begin to understand about the joy of womanhood and that menstruation will play a role in her becoming a mother one day, insha'Allah. We women must take advantage of our periods, use them to rest and reflect inwardly, and simply accept that the body is cleansing itself. If we ourselves have a good relationship with our bodies, so will our daughters.

Premenstrual syndrome (PMS)

Menstruation is a physiological process that should not be problematic or painful. Pain could be due to a mild dysfunction that may disappear with osteopathy or homoeopathy, but a doctor should be consulted if the problem persists.

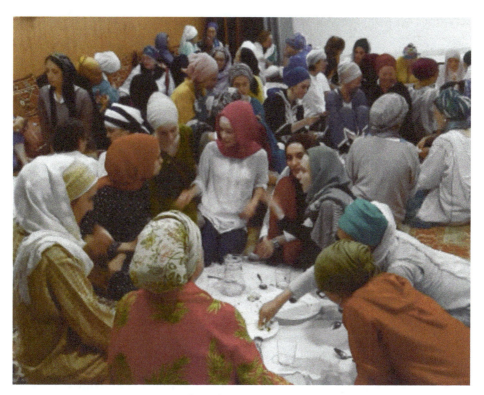

However, even in a normal cycle, we notice hormonal fluctuations that occur in the first and second part of the cycle and cause physiological and emotional changes in us. Oestrogen dominates the first half of the menstrual cycle before ovulation and boosts self-confidence, positive energy and immunity; while progesterone dominates during the second half and prepares the endometrium to receive a fertilised egg. Progesterone also lowers the body's immune defences, which is why we sometimes come down with a cold or get cystitis just before our period.

PMS is triggered by an imbalance between oestrogen and progesterone levels, simply because in the second half of the cycle, the level of progesterone is relatively lower than that of oestrogen and is insufficient to counteract the oestrogen.

Oestrogen has a pro-inflammatory effect and causes bloating, water retention and breast tenderness, while progesterone produces calmness but can cause irritability if there is not enough of it.

We can moderate these effects by eating an anti-inflammatory diet with a good balance of omega-3 (linseed/flaxseed, chia seed, nuts, oily fish) and omega-6 (butter, red meat), in correct proportions. Turmeric and pepper can also help, and above all avoiding animal hormones passed on through milk and ingesting bisphenols (such as BPA), which can leach out of plastic containers into food and drink.

Pregnancy

When we get pregnant, rather than treating it as an illness we should enjoy the happy, contemplative, dreamy state that we may be experiencing.

Facing a new situation can also make us feel scared and insecure, so it is very important to feel protected and supported by our husband and family, as well as the community of women. Knowing that we can count on the women around us creates

> *Obviously, raising a child well, without going mad, is very difficult when you are alone in a flat, isolated in a nuclear family!*

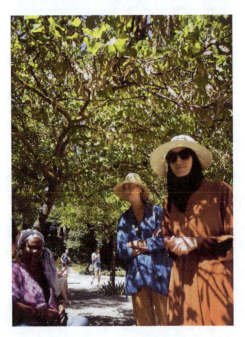

trust and reduces stress and fear, which helps correct foetal development and increases the likelihood of a natural labour.

The mother-to-be should avoid stress as much as possible and uplift herself with good thoughts, sounds and beautiful views of nature to generate endorphins that reach the baby.

On a more physical level, she should take care with her diet by avoiding large oily fish, which contain mercury (a neurotoxin), and processed foods full of salt, sugar and preservatives, and eat natural food full of life-giving energy instead of empty calories. It is also recommendable to go for walks and do gentle physical exercise, such as yoga, Pilates or tai chi, but not to the point of exhaustion. Exercises seated on a Pilates ball should only be done from the seventh month of pregnancy because the vibration softens the cervix.

When it comes to labour, mind-body techniques focused on breathing can lessen the pain of contractions and ease childbirth, and the support of wise and experienced women will also help. But, first and foremost, it is trust in Allah instead of in techniques that gives a woman the necessary strength and determination to make her labour her own and bring her baby into the world in the most natural way possible.

I still remember giving birth to my second child at home. I was accompanied by two Muslim women doing dhikr (we are forever bonded as sisters), while my husband supported us with *du'a*, as he waited in the next room to receive the baby and call the *adhan*.

Knowing that Allah is taking care of us and that He will give us what is best enables us to accept the outcome. It is important not to get stressed because stress raises the level of cortisol, a hormone that increases the likelihood of premature labour, low birth weight and decreased attention in infancy. Even so, the new mother should not worry because her love and dedication during the immediate postpartum period will help the newborn gain weight quickly. Through breastfeeding, she will pass antibodies and endorphins on to the baby, as well as oxytocin (the "love hormone"). Oxytocin helps to create a secure mother–child bond by producing empathy and love between mother and child. Together with prolactin, it also increases the

Epigenetics describes how acquired characteristics can be transmitted to offspring via chemical markers that cause some genes to activate but others not. This is effected through diet, habits, stress, behaviour and even meditation (techniques we would call dhikr in our circles).

milk supply and boosts the mother's motivation to protect the baby, thereby encouraging lactation. In turn, breastfeeding and endorphins protect against postnatal depression.

In the first six weeks after the birth, the mother's sole concern should be the baby. Delighted with her little bundle of joy but tired, she must allow herself to be looked after, delegate to others and rely on the women around her to cook restorative soups and do the other tasks. Even if the new mother feels well, remember that not only has the uterus expanded, but relaxin (a hormone secreted by the placenta) has reached all the joints by this time and they are now much more vulnerable to cold, so it is essential to keep warm. Spending those first 40 days at home with the baby is not an insignificant or old-fashioned practice – we must respect it in order to avoid getting ill. The support and advice of the women around her helps the mother with breastfeeding and makes her feel safe and secure in the knowledge that she is protected.

Pelvic floor recovery

During childbirth, it is very normal for the pelvic floor to stretch or even tear a little, or to have been cut during an episiotomy. This should all be checked by a professional. The pelvic floor is 70% fibrous tissue and can become damaged during birth if it is overstretched. Scarring may be painful and can be treated with creams and massages to restore elasticity. Short massages of the perineal area can be done during pregnancy to make it more elastic for labour. Do not simply accept pain as something normal, because it may lead to problems later on during the menopause.

From three months after giving birth, you can start doing hypopressive and Kegel exercises to re-strengthen the pelvic floor. Do not think about trying to regain your figure before this time, as doing abdominal exercises like crunches only increases the pressure on the pelvic floor and exacerbates any problems.

It is important to strengthen the pelvic floor after giving birth because it weakens during menopause as a result of the drop in oestrogen, and any untreated issues will worsen. Even if you had a completely natural labour, if you later notice any symptoms of incontinence when exerting yourself, do not ignore them because they can return during the menopause.

Epigenetics

Epigenetics is important in understanding how we can influence our health and that of future generations, which is something that we're concerned with when we are pregnant.

We always think of genes as fixed and unchanging, but they are not entirely so. In the 18th Century, the French biologist Jean-Baptiste Lamarck argued the theory of the inheritance of acquired characteristics. That same century, despite having been initially rejected, his theory was proven true through epigenetics.

Epigenetics describes how acquired characteristics can be transmitted to offspring via chemical markers that cause some

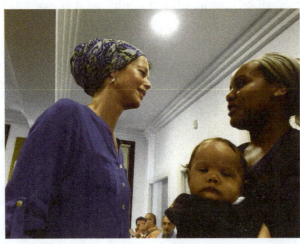

genes to activate but others not. This is effected through diet, habits, stress, behaviour and even meditation (techniques we would call dhikr in our circles). These changes can be transmitted to offspring, influencing the genes and the epigenome. Consequently, adults who were raised with a secure attachment bond to their parents will be able to transmit the benefit of that secure attachment when bringing up their own children, passing it down through the generations.

Child-rearing and attachment

The mother's attitude from the moment the child is born and during the first two years is critical. Forming a secure attachment enables the child to establish healthy relationships with other people, including the choice of a good spouse and creation of a sounder society – that goes for men and women. Therefore, women, as child-rearers, are already promoting the health of future generations.

The theory of attachment was created by the psychiatrist John Bowlby, who conducted studies in the 1950s of children orphaned by the Second World War. He argued that a healthy, lasting and warm mother–child relationship gave pleasure to both parties and allowed the baby to be raised with secure attachment. The mother transmits not only care for the child's basic needs, but also takes care of its emotional needs and sense of security, something that enables the child to have good self-esteem and establish healthy relationships in the future. And if the baby is a girl, it is obvious how essential it is to transmit that secure attachment to her, in particular, as a future mother.

There are four types of attachment:

Secure attachment:

As previously explained, this type of attachment enables the child to become an independent person who does not feel anxiety when alone.

Anxious–ambivalent attachment:

The mother is sometimes present and sometimes not, which makes the child feel insecure when exploring the world, leading to emotional dependence in later life.

Avoidant attachment:

The child learns not to rely on the carers and seems to be a good and independent child. In fact, he or she simply has no expectations.

Disorganised attachment:

The worst and least frequent of the four types, it is a mixture of anxious attachment and avoidant attachment. It generally results from abuse and leads to explosive behaviour in the future.

Again, we should not worry too much. Obviously, raising a child well, without going mad, is very difficult when you are alone in a flat, isolated in a nuclear family! It takes a whole tribe to raise a child, and the support of that tribe is also important for the physical and emotional health of the mother.

Those who are not mothers can use their creativity and artistic talents to express the mercy inherent in womankind. Even if you are not creative, you can show that mercy by caring for other members of our community: neighbours' children, nieces and nephews, grandchildren or whoever needs your help and knowledge.

> *Market interests have contaminated everything to do with women's life processes and sexuality: they are selling us youth.*

Giving to other women is just as beneficial as receiving. When we reach the menopause and probably have more time on our hands, it is a good idea to give back.

Menopause

The menopause is not an illness. It is just the end of the reproductive phase of a woman's life, lasting some 40 years. Naturally, it is difficult to say goodbye to such a long and significant part of our lives, but we as Muslims know that life is a constant change and that, with this new phase, perhaps we will finally have some time for ourselves.

The menopause does not happen all of a sudden but begins with shorter, lighter menstrual cycles that then become less frequent. Treatment should only be sought if there is haemorrhaging. Depending on whether we see this stage as a loss and on how we have lived before, emotional symptoms may accompany the physical ones. If we medicate these changes, we will miss out on the chance to grow and understand that we are entering that second part of our lives which involves greater self-reflection, spirituality and dhikr. We should take advantage of opportunities to cultivate our knowledge at this time and also throughout our lives – because wisdom does not come just with age – and apply it in our communities and even in what we do with our grandchildren.

In terms of exercise, one of the best practices is to get some sun by

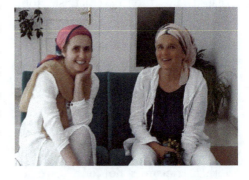

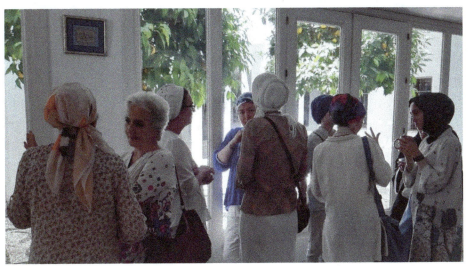

walking outdoors. Aerobics and a little light weightlifting help to combat osteoporosis, and a healthy diet helps to conserve energy. Above all, having a life project to fulfil will increase our lust for life. Holistic exercises that improve body awareness and balance, like yoga and tai chi, re-energise us and help us to know ourselves.

Conclusion

I want to emphasise that, as Muslim women, we must accept change, remembering that things in life are impermanent and in a state of flux. Ageing is wonderful when you don't allow yourself to be swayed by this society's myths of eternal youth and eternal energy. Market interests have contaminated everything to do with women's life processes and sexuality: they are selling us youth.

With Allah's permission, we hold in our hands a great part of the responsibility for our health. He has given us a body to take care of, which we must return one day, together with a life energy that will last us for a longer or shorter time, depending on how we treat it. This energy will allow us to live full lives, insha'Allah, and if that is not the case, we must accept the light and the dark of life, because without the darkness, we cannot appreciate the light. We must not pretend that life is a bed of roses and wish for a knight in shining armour to come and rescue us. We must be active, full and open to experience and teaching so that we can become strong women with enough emotional intelligence to be able to choose a good companion to accompany us on the unfolding of our mutual life journey within the deen. Ameen.

Human beings cannot be alone. Attachment to other people is vital, just like the basic needs for food and sex. If you are alone, you don't talk; if you don't talk, you dream about your worries, and if you don't dream about them, you somatise them and they manifest in the body as illnesses, muscle pains, anxiety and so on.

Social relationships are healing. When we women talk among ourselves, we share the burden of daily life. Talking and sharing can lighten the load and show you that you are not the only one with doubts or going through a rough patch. We can then look objectively at things and even laugh together. The problems diminish, and when we have no problems and think positively, we can create projects together, just as we are doing right here, right now.

TAHIRA NARBONA

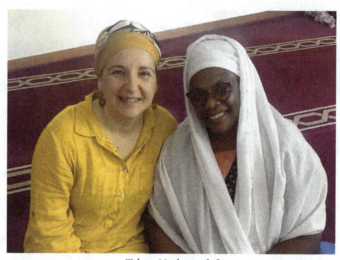

Tahira Narbona (left)

Democratic Tyranny and the Islamic Paradigm
An Introduction

This talk, based on the book of the same name, served as a springboard to beginning a discussion around alternatives to governance and social welfare.

I don't know how many of you have read the book, but today we are basically going to be discussing a few future ideas; I am not going to go over the philosophy of the book which is chiefly concerned with the origins of democracy and the fact that what goes by the term "democracy" now is the idea of the rule by the people. But "democracy" is not really the rule of the people. Even if you have a referendum where everybody votes, it is all set up by the amount of information the people are given. And who gives you that information? Who tells you what's a good idea to vote on? Generally, it is people in the media, who have their own financial concerns — so you are never going to get a "balanced" view in order to make a balanced decision.

It even comes down to the question and the form of the question you are asked. And the Internet has made this worse. One of the things I mention in the book is Shoshana Zuboff's text, *The Age of Surveillance Capitalism*. The questions Zuboff poses throughout the book are:

Who knows?

Who decides?

Who decides who decides?

Here, the answer is *not* the general populace, it isn't the people.

Now there's another point that's been written about a lot these days and that is that we may be approaching the end of the nation state. It is only three hundred years old. But you would have noticed that populism and quasi-totalitarian kind of leaders are on the rise. We have Trump in America, we have Kaczyński in Poland, Salvini in Italy, Orbán in Hungary, Putin in Russia and so on. Plato said that "Democracy always ends in totalitarian rule," and is done through security. They make you afraid and say: "You need extra measures to make you safe!" As these measures increase, you lose more and more of your freedoms.

We are in a very interesting period, because, as I said before, it's a time of flux — it's a time of change. Churchill said: "Democracy is terrible. But it's the best of what's available." We have something better, and what we have hasn't been tried.

Granada, Spain, June 2019

This is why I've outlined some of the details in the book – but we cannot snap our fingers and have it come into being. The most recent example of an alternative is the Caliphate in Kano, Northern Nigeria, which is still in existence, but there are attempts to have its power completely eliminated. That's the most recent example of someone trying to implement a form of this other type of governance. What is interesting is the way they chose a ruler – they didn't necessarily pick the son of the ruler. Instead, all the people of the household who had any degree of standing were considered as candidates. Then certain people such as the imams, the generals, the people who were high ministers in the government, met, and decided who would be the best ruler from that group of people. So it wasn't a pure democracy of everybody voting, but there was a level of democracy, a level of selection. People who were not part of this process could, however, come forward and make statements and representations, so there was participation.

This is what is facing us, we need ideas and we need suggestions – and we may come up with new ideas. Do you know where the idea of the jury came from – the twelve men who judge a case in court? It came from the Muslims! There was a period in England called the Anarchy, during the early Plantagenet period in which the Empress Matilda and her cousin Stephan fought. Everything got destroyed, all the forms of government. Finally, they decided that since Stephan's only son had died, Matilda's son would be the king after Stephan. He became Henry II and said: "We're in a mess. Everything is destroyed." So he turned to a man who was called Qaid Brun, whose original name was Thomas Brown and who had been in Sicily. Some of the Plantagenets were in Sicily for a while, and he was Roger's treasurer there becoming intimately acquainted with Muslim law. And Henry said to him: "Fix everything!"

In Islam, to be a witness you have to reach a certain level of character and at this stage in Morocco it was felt that no one met this requirement anymore. So they decided that due to the deficiencies in character, they would use twelve people instead. And that is the origin of the jury. This is just one example.

When you find that you're living in a society in which you don't have everything that you need, you have to come with new ideas and new

> *Plato said that "Democracy always ends in totalitarian rule," and is done through security.*

suggestions. We have to start small. We have to have a leader who collects zakat and gives it to the people, to begin building a kind of unity. But we need more than this. So… ideas!

Aisha Bewley

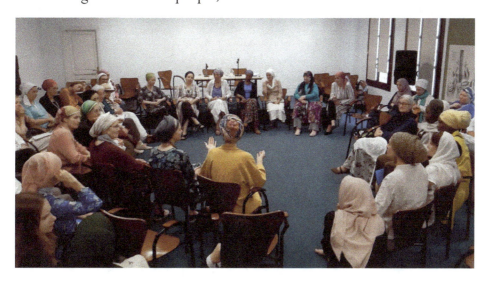

SOCIAL WELFARE BEYOND THE STATE: ESTABLISHING AWQAF

I want to begin first by talking about our possibilities as women and why the awqaf are a vital aspect of resistance in this time and then highlight the more technical pre-requisites of establishing a waqf.

As men and women, we have different responsibilities, different inherent qualities and different needs, but the heart of a community is the women. Allah ta'ala, has put within us an organ which is unique to us, which defines the nature of the woman. This is the womb, which in Arabic is *rahm*, which comes from *rahma*, mercy. This is a hidden gift and it is no accident that women are being shamed out of being mothers and expected to go out into the male sphere, where they lose this inherent quality in an increasingly aggressive and macho world.

Whilst the men are more typically engaged in furthering the realm of authority, trade and business, in all traditional and *fitra* societies it is the women who maintain the community and continue to keep it functioning. Both aspects are vital to the full and complete functioning of the community. It is often the case that the women cater for the more grassroots and practical needs. This results in us having a deeper, mutual connection that arises out of daily life, such as looking after each other's children, and it is how we begin to share our difficulties and ease.

We currently live in a world that has been designed by men, or proxy men: the banking system, the Internet, the iPhone, Amazon, Google and Facebook are all creations of a male approach of conquering and dominating. It is this approach and intense yearning for power and domination that is killing the human being. It is necessary to look at the character of the people who have created the world in which we live, because, as Ibn al-Arabi said, we create a model of existence that reflects ourself. The proof of this is found in the creation of the city of lights, Madinah al Munawara whose founder was the perfect human, the Prophet Muhammad ﷺ.

In this age, we must accept that there is a vacuum of genuine feminine power. And as Shaykh Abdalqadir as-Sufi said at his inaugural talk at the Lady Aisha College:

> *In this age we must accept that there is a vacuum of genuine feminine power.*

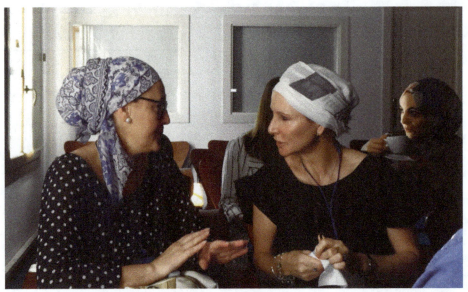

Rahima Brandt, right, in conversation with a conference attendee

"... One has to realise that power is responsibility and pretending that women do not have power is a lie against natural life... [the College] is simply a means for women to study how they can survive the appalling world that men have made for themselves and for us, how they can survive it without turning into them, as matriarchs, begums and dominant destroying forces of more terrible power than the men have."

It is therefore clear that as women, it is up to us to engage with our feminine power and to return compassion and mercy to the incredibly difficult age in which we are living.

Allah ta'ala, has given us a Deen, which puts in place a way of living that protects the human being, *if* we put it into place. It is tangible and defies the usurious system that makes people slaves. It is based on *assabiya*, genuine care and concern for the Ummah. Crucial aspects of the Deen in addition to the obligatory *zakat* are the *sadaqa* and the *awqaf*, which are necessary to maintain and strengthen the fabric of society, and are always the result of the *mu'minun* who have *taqwa*, and hearts that are alive and seeing the needs of the people around them. It begins with personal responsibility and accountability.

What I hope to do here is to open up what possibilities we might have to start grassroots activities which can benefit us all, give life to our Deen and indeed to assist humanity as a whole. In order to do this, I would like to give a simple overview of the purpose of the awqaf system and the parameters that guide its setting up and continuation. My goal is to make it as practical as possible and to share with you some examples of how simple setting up a waqf can be.

In its essence, the waqf is basically a way of looking after the community, which renders the state apparatus unnecessary. It is from the people for the people. It completely removes the need for state interference, and it is by this means that the community looks after itself. It encourages the community to have an overview of itself and to become responsible for the needs of one another. The setting up of awqaf, following the establishment of the mosque and the marketplace are the beginning of a properly functioning community as it addresses the primary needs of the community. Furthermore, there are certain awqaf that exist in perpetuity, so that the *baraka* of this sadaqa reaches beyond the grave.

The first person to set up a waqf was the Rasul ﷺ. Once he had established the mosque in Madinah, he established the marketplace, which remains a waqf to this day. All the Companions of the Prophet ﷺ who had any means established awqaf and they were set up to address the most pressing needs of the time. In order to set up a waqf, there must be a functioning economy and Shaykh Habib Bewley recently reminded us that nine out of ten of the Companions promised the Garden were traders — the exception being Sayyiduna Ali who was too young.

Abdarrahman ibn Awf, who was one of these Companions promised the Garden, was a trader who in today's terms was probably a number of times wealthier than Bill Gates. When he died he left 4000 Dirhams to every single Badri (fighter in Badr). Remember, too that this was only from the one third of the estate that you are allowed to bequeath.

Shaykh Habib went on to explain that although these men were wealthy and they traded, they were not too busy to stop and help their community. It is this spirit, of doing business with the aim of having the resources to set up awqaf for the benefit of others, that is a noble and high aspiration. It also enables

> *In its essence, the waqf is basically a way of looking after the community, which renders the state apparatus unnecessary. (...) It encourages the community to have an overview of itself and to become responsible for the needs of one another.*

us to look upon our work with a completely different outlook of excitement and joy at the possibility of being able to contribute to raising up and strengthening the deen of Islam.

Awqaf have always been set up to address the pressing needs of the time first and we find many examples of this taking place. During a time of drought, Sayyiduna Uthman gave a well as a waqf; and when they were engaged in jihad, Sayyiduna Umar gave horses as a waqf for soldiers who did not have a horse. There was another waqf, which was basically a pasture where the horses grazed when they weren't fighting. In times of war, there were awqaf for the widows. So, awqaf have been set up for many things: mosques, hospitals, water sources, but also streets, bridges, graveyards, modes of transports, boats — the list is endless. In Istanbul, under Ottoman rule, the awqaf were so numerous that there

were even awqaf to feed the birds.

The definition of a waqf according to Imam Malik, is to give the benefits of something, and for it to be limited to those for whom it is delineated. This means that you can have a property which is a waqf and the use of that property could, for example, be solely for the use of newlyweds who have no home. Or the income from renting out the property could be given to the newlyweds. The recipient would always be newlyweds, so this is an example of

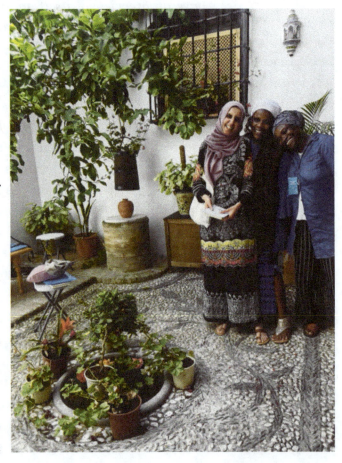

limiting who is able to use it based on a primary need.

The parameters of establishing a waqf are the following:

The first parameter is that the recipients of the waqf must be clearly defined. It could be, for example, only for those who ordinarily receive zakat, or for the elderly who have no family or for the members of a particular family. It must be clearly defined, so that there is no contention over the beneficiaries. In fact, the modern-day trusts that people set up for their families originally came from the awqaf.

The second parameter is that it must be a specific item or known quantity, which is dedicated to the waqf. So, you can't say "I give everything I have in my shed for a waqf", if you don't know exactly what you have in your shed. The length of time of the waqf's existence must also be known. It is best that it is forever, but according to Imam Malik, it can also be for a stipulated period of time, after which the original elements of the waqf return to the person who set it up. However, it should be clear when it is established what the time period is, otherwise it is assumed that is forever and it cannot be disbanded.

> *It is this spirit, of doing business with the aim of having the resources to set up awqaf for the benefit of others, that is a noble and high aspiration.*

The waqf can also be set up for as long as the commodity, which provides the income, is functioning. So, it could be a horse, which provides transport, but obviously the horse will eventually die. You could have a car, which is a taxi and the income from that is used for the specified recipients of the waqf, but when that car no longer works, the waqf would end. The important aspect here is that you can do something small. It is possible to start without having to have an enormous amount of wealth.

A waqf can be property from which income is earned, it could be a car, a business, basically anything that produces an income or provides a service. Of course, it can be the property or land itself – Sayyiduna Umar was given land when they conquered Khaybar and he divided it out and made each one a waqf. But it can also be the fruits of the land. In the time of the Rasul ﷺ orchards were given or even just the fruits from the trees in the orchards.

Awqaf can also consist of commodities. For example, you could have a grain store, which is a waqf and those people who are the delineated beneficiaries of that waqf are given grain when they need it. Equally, they can give back that grain to the waqf when they are in better circumstances, should they choose.

The waqf can also be a place of lending. For example, you could have money in the waqf which is loaned interest-free to people who need it for businesses or pressing needs. Years ago, I had a rocking chair and as my children were grown up, I didn't need it anymore. I gave it to a friend of mine who had just had a baby and I said her: "When you finish with it, give it to the next person who has a baby." So, this chair went from mother to mother to mother, but somewhere along the way it disappeared. It turns out that even this rocking chair could have been established as a waqf! By establishing it as a waqf, there would have been greater responsibility and accountability and there would be more baraka in it, and probably it wouldn't have disappeared!

It is also possible to start a business or have a business of which you make a percentage a waqf, for example, whereby 50% of the profits are a waqf, (but the waqf is not respon-

sible for the losses of the business). Although awqaf were typically set up by individuals, they can also be set up by groups of people.

The further conditions of a Waqf are the following:

The person endowing it must be Muslim, they must either own the object which is to be the waqf or they must have the full benefit of it. If, for example, you are renting a building and you have a long lease, you can set up a waqf for a specific time period in which you rent it as an AirBnB and the profits of that short rental is for the waqf – so long as during this time you have the full benefit of the building as the long-term lessee.

The second condition is that the person setting it up must be what is called *rashid*, someone who is sound in finances. It cannot be done by someone who is *safih*, someone who has no sense of financial responsibility and is not sound in finances. Such a person, if they want to establish a waqf can do so with the help of a designated guardian.

The waqf also requires an administrator and they will have a wage for whatever they do for the waqf. Shaykh Habib also said that it is best that the person who sets up the waqf does not run the waqf, in order to ensure that the waqf is not used for purposes of power and reputation.

In addition to paying the administrator a salary, you must also consider the cost of maintaining the waqf, such as the maintenance of a building, cleaning, feeding the horse and so on.

So, who can be the beneficiary of a waqf?

It can be specific people or even people who are not yet born, or it can be used to support the running of an entity, a hospital, centre or school. The recipients don't have to be Muslims, so long as they fulfill the conditions of the waqf. In other words, if a waqf has been designated for widows, then the beneficiary or recipient only has to fulfill that requirement of being a widow.

Finally, it is considered that it is best to set up a waqf whilst you are alive, as opposed to leaving it in an inheritance. This is because when you are well, it is so much harder to cleave yourself of your wealth, so there is more baraka and benefit for you in it. The Prophet 𐍈 said:

> *The important aspect here is that you can do something small. It is possible to start without having to have an enormous amount of wealth.*

"*A person giving a single Dirham when he is alive and in a good health is better than giving a hundred Dirhams when he is on the point of dying.*"

It is also important to remember the Ayat of Qur'an where Allah ta'ala says "*Shaytan promises you poverty*". Shaytan whispers that to you, to try to prevent you from giving by provoking fear of provision, to stop you putting in place the Deen.

I want to leave you by reminding you that a waqf can be something small. It is better to start with what we have, rather than have too lofty aspirations, which prevent us from putting it in place. By setting up small awqaf within our current capabilities, we open the door for more baraka, and inshallah, open the way to take on a greater and greater capacity to look after each other. On intention, great things are grown.

May Allah ta'ala make us people of awqaf and give us the means so that we have the capacity to create a complete and vibrant community, fully enacting the Sunna of our beloved Messenger 𐍈.

Postcript 2020

In the light of the covid-19 'crisis' and the exposed weaknesses of modern global corporative governance to resolve the fundamental issues of poverty and community connection, it has never been more important to put in place the revealed social welfare aspects of the deen. Localisation of economy, caring for your neighbours, freedom to trade without taxes and reinvesting in your community are all fundamental to the flourishing of the deen. The awqaf is one tool in the kit which is supported by the local collection and distribution of zakat, the establishment of local markets with no fees for sellers and the restoration of the guilds to nurture young talent. The regeneration of society will need these measures to be established more now than ever.

RAHIMA BRANDT

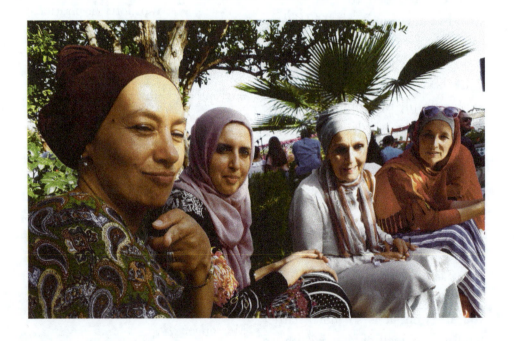

The Importance of Guarding the Heart

I think we all agree that the last few days have been an enormous success, days of deep inspiration, renewal and such a reminder of the great gift we have been given which we must treasure and hold firm in our hearts.

We spoke much on the differences between men and women, but of course in the Batin, in the Inward, there is no difference – in the matter of Taqwa.

I think we all know the meaning of Taqwa. We can say it is "guarding yourself", or "being careful". Perhaps you could use the analogy of how the lover is with their beloved. When you are in love, you are careful, very careful because you want to be pleasing, you are fearful that the beloved will be displeased with you, so are careful what you say, careful in your actions and so on. This is how we want to be with our Lord; we love Allah therefore we must be careful. Quran: "...*The end of the affair is for the people of Taqwa.*"

The Prophet ﷺ said: "Taqwa is here" as he pointed to his heart. The heart is the home of all inner qualities.

As we know, this path we are on is about the purification of the heart. So let us remind ourselves a little about the nature of the heart. Shaykh Mohammed ibn al-Habib says in The Great Ode in his Diwan: "A man would not hesitate to spend everything he had if he only understood the secret of his own heart. If a man would grasp the bliss of his secret he would shed a tear with every breath he breathed". If we take these words seriously and reflect on them – what a mighty thing – and surely this is what we want. These words we must reflect on and literally take to heart.

It is on returning to our everyday lives after such a wonderful event that we have to be particularly careful in guarding our hearts, coupled with what we see happening in the world around us. In the coming world which we see is breaking up so fast on every level, our primary task is to guard, protect and nourish our hearts, this extraordinary organ, which is continually in flux, continually moving from one state to another state, responding to what the eye falls on, responding to what the ear hears, responding to what the senses feel. Shaykh Abdalqadir once said that the physical heart and the ruhaani heart are not separate, for this reason you may have organ transplants but never a heart transplant.

Scientists are now discovering fascinating things about the heart: apparently it is not just the brain sending messages to the body but the heart actually sends messages to the brain. Shaykh Abdalqadir in his book *The Way of Muhammad*, refers several times to quantum physics, he says that he refers to it not as proof but as a way to help us understand, so if I may I am going to refer to what I have been reading about from the quantum physicists. And please, if I am wrong about this, Aisha Bewley who knows a great deal about this matter, do put me right. These physicists are using the word 'entanglement' and in their description of this they are saying that the whole world is one thing and we are part of it. What we are doing and what the world is doing are intimately coupled. There is no such thing as me doing something independently of the world, and no such thing as the world doing something independently of me. Everything is like a mirror. Shaykh Abdalqadir describes this when he is talking of Rububiyyat – Lordship: "the interconnectedness of all things,

> *I recognise that over the years some of us have been hurt, pained or disappointed. Things happen. This is reflected in the heart. The danger here is that unless we consciously let go, this can harden the heart. Yet the heart is all we really own.*

all events, all creatures are connected in the web of Rububiyyat'. It is the same with our hearts, our hearts are not in isolation, every thought, every state we have is not in isolation, every thought and action is connected and has an effect. Shaykh Abdalqadir once described the heart as being fought over between the light of the Ruh and the darkness of the Self. The real function of the heart is to mirror the light of Allah, because we are not dark beings, our reality is a locus of light, but our hearts are obscured by the cloudiness of our thoughts. This cloudiness is of course dispelled by dhikrAllah. See how after gatherings of dhikr the light shows on our faces! It is visible.

The Prophet ﷺ said "Truly in the body there is a piece of flesh which, when it is sound the whole body is sound, and when it is diseased the whole body is diseased. And it is the heart". Ibn Ajiba says, "The son of Adam is created of two worlds, the subtle and the solid....The heart is like a mirror". Everything is imprinted on the heart.

Everything since the day we were born is imprinted on our hearts. It is said that at the end of life the whole of one's life flashes by before one's eyes. Perhaps many of us have tasted this in that barzakh-state on falling asleep, when suddenly an ancient long forgotten memory pops up from nowhere as if it had happened yesterday.

Therefore, we have to guard our hearts. I recognise that over the years some of us have been hurt, pained or disappointed, things happen. This is reflected in the heart. The danger here is that unless we consciously let go, this can harden the heart. Yet the heart is all we really own. I often reflect that the one thing to be fearful of is to die with a bitter or hard heart. But how many prophets, how many walis, how many great people of Allah had far greater wrongs done to them than what we have ever had. They were rejected, betrayed, misunderstood, thrown out, but they guarded their hearts. They guarded their hearts! They did not separate.

Allah is closer to you than your jugular vein. He is Qarib, He is closer than life itself. He is the Merciful. In the hadith qudsi Allah ta'ala says "I am in My slave's opinion of Me". We say with our tongues Allah ta'ala is Merciful, but what is the reality of our thinking? There can be an enormous gap between what we say and what we think. So what is the reality of our opinion of Allah ta'ala? All of us have times of constriction, but if we have long, ongoing, negative thought patterns, then we are not having good opinion of Allah. We can also call up events equal to our thoughts, because Allah is in our opinion of Him. Allah ta'ala is al-Haqq. He is the Real — our reality.

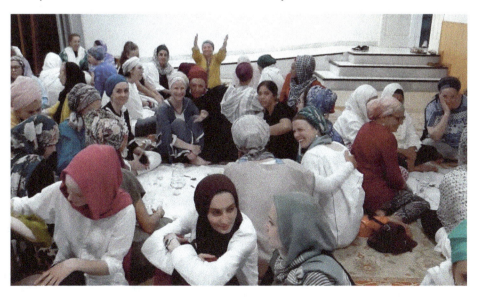

If you will excuse me, I want to refer to quantum physics again (I suggest you read, if interested, Aisha's book, *Subatomic World in the Quran*). Quantum Physics says that matter, on an energetic level, is 99.99999% nothing – no thing. Empty space consisting of energy waves which carry information. Shaykh Abdalqadir puts it this way: "The reality of this great, vast myriad world of creation is a nothingness on which is sustained this tremendous event of creation, man himself is a vibrating, whirling activity of energy in endless movement." Shaykh Mohammed ibn al Habib says in his diwan, "I tore down the illusion of myself and found Him timeless in every atom". To return again to quantum physics: the solid material of the classical physicists dissolves into wave like probabilities. Shaykh Abdalqadir puts it this way: "We are not wandering in a desert, but living through a situation where everything is alive and full of possibilities".

So we have this language: probabilities, possibilities. Everything is possible with Allah. But remember "Allah is in your opinion of Him'.

> *You are calling on the One Who knows you better than anyone else, better than you know yourself. And He is the Merciful. We forget and remember, forget and remember. Turn back, turn back, a thousand times turn back, as Rumi says.*

In this perhaps rather complicated fashion of putting this matter, what I am attempting to say in simple terms is – if we have difficult times with ourselves, with our thought patternings – if we wish, we can change. But we cannot change ourselves through our selves as Shaykh Abdalqadir says in *The Way of Muhammad*: "You cannot think or detector-feel your way out of the contradictions and pains of life's existence". Neither can we say to ourselves 'I must be more…..." or "I should be more…..". For this is Christianity, and thinking we are in charge. For instance let us look at the stories in the Quran of Sayedina Musa ﷺ who, it is mentioned, was often fearful. He was a human being with all the fears we have. There are many times when he says "Ya Allah, I am fearful". He is fearful lest he be killed or that the people will not understand him and more. He is not saying "I must not be afraid". No, he is handing his fear over to His Lord, he is handing it over. This is dhikrullah. As Shaykh Mohammed ibn al Habib says "The rewards of dhikr are without limit".

I have heard many people say dhikr does not work like it is a magic pill, yet when we are stuck in a corner and there is no where else to go, no one to turn to, we all say "Allah". We need to remember Him as much as we can because we are talking about the heart, about the difficulties of the heart, the thoughts that veil our hearts. And there is nothing, there is nothing that cuts through the thoughts and the veils over the heart better than dhikrullah. You are calling on the One Who knows you better than anyone else, better than you know yourself. And He is the Merciful. We forget and remember, forget and remember. Turn back, turn back, a thousand times turn back, as Rumi says. We either have remembrance of ourselves or remembrance of Allah and remembrance of ourselves brings us nothing but trouble.

...it may not be the age to go into seclusion and do vast amounts of dhikr, it certainly is an age that calls for action. But action done WITH dhikr will have a very different result.

There is a secret to dhikrullah and that is that when you call, you are calling with longing, with yearning, with your whole being. "Make all your worries one" as Shaykh Mohammed ibn al Habib says. All our fears, doubts and matters we have in the heart, turn them over, knowing,

knowing that He will answer you. As the Prophet ﷺ said, "When you call on your Lord, call with a will."

There are many people I have heard say that it is not the time to do dhikr, it is not the age to do dhikr. In part this is true, it may not be the age to go into seclusion and do vast amounts of dhikr, it certainly is an age that calls for action. But action done WITH dhikr will have a very different result.

We see all the terrible injustices that are happening in the world, we gather together and call for justice, turning to La ilaha illAllah in our hearts.

We know there are difficulties within the communities where we must take action and join hearts with kindness, as in the hadith "Allah is Kind and loves kindness in all things, and confers upon kindness that which He does not confer upon anything besides it." Also, "He who is deprived of kindness is deprived of goodness". We help each other and return to La ilaha illAllah in our hearts.

When we have difficulties with ourselves, turbulent times, we turn to La ilaha illAllah again and again and again.

Finally, since I have mentioned frequently the hadith qudsi: "I am in your opinion of Me". Allah ta'ala is in our opinion of Him. So we must remember He is al-Lateef, al-Khabir. Shaykh Abdalqadir commenting on these two names of Allah says, "The meaning of Lateef is graciousness and kindness, also of penetrating right through everything, pervasive but with infinite kindness and closeness. Khabir is total awareness that takes in everything, all the time. That is how we must understand Allah ta'ala all the time."

This is good opinion.

Salat an-Nabi

Fatiha

RABEA REDPATH

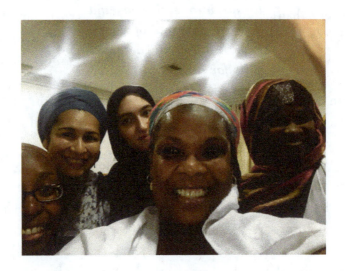

Conclusions of the Women's Conference

I would like to thank you for allowing me the opportunity to talk at the anniversary of the Great Mosque of Granada and share important reflections from the very first Women's Encounters Conference.

When I arrived in Granada, the first thing I saw upon getting off the bus was a massive poster advertising an exhibition of the torture instruments used during the Spanish Inquisition. I began to reflect on the significance of the conference being hosted in this city and I began to think about some of the history, so if you will permit me – I would like to dig into some of your history.

The final conquest of Al-Andalus in the late 15th century destroyed the sultanate of Granada, which was the last Muslim political authority on the Iberian Peninsula. To succeed, there needed to be a physical genocide, that is to say selective torture and killings culminating in a full expulsion. Additionally, there needed to be a cultural genocide, that is to say the destruction of Islamic knowledge and spirituality through forced conversions. The cultural genocide ensured that the descendants of *moriscos* would be born without any memory to trace their ancestors.

The Castillan monarchy did not simply seek to rule the territory, but it enacted a system which became the blueprint for genocides and epistimicides that have shaped modernity. Simply put, it was the idea of "one state, one identity, one religion" – an idea which is gaining more and more traction the world over in some form or another. This was in direct contrast to Al-Andalus with its multiplicities, it's knowledge centers in which there was a free exchange of thoughts and ideas, recognition and respect for multiple identities, as well as the guarantee of rights granted to Jews and Christians and the system of the *jizya* tax. This is how the Muslims governed in Granada, and so it is in this city that we witness an early example of a transition from government to "governmentality". Or, to use the language of *The Entire City*, it is to move from "the governance of men to the administration of things". The identity of the state had to be superimposed on the identity of the population.

The Castillan monarchy wanted to achieve three things:
control
surveillance
homogeneity

GRANADA, SPAIN, JUNE 2019

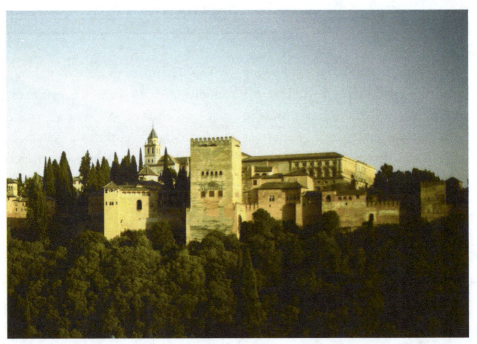

It is tempting to draw striking parallels to the present day, but for the time being I would like to highlight that it is this aspect of homogeneity or homogenous thought which is a key aspect to the functioning of the modern state. The dullness of conformity and the lack of space for dissent is something which we are confronted with today. We are taught to think alike, act alike and reduce all our behavior to the lowest common denominator. We are taught that we must agree on the same things and disagree on the same things. There is no space for nuance. There is no space to question. Why? Because if sameness can be achieved, it means that every person's actions and reactions can be predicted.

Thus, this gathering of women is a break with homogenous thought. It is a break with the "sameness". It is an opportunity to gather the perceptions of women and the ideas of women and the thoughts of women as a group in order to declare: "No. We are not the same. We are different." Therefore, it should immediately be clear that we are not embarking on the kind of feminist project which reduces men and women to one entity. Instead we are saying: "We are different, we have different needs and different priorities. We may even come up with different solutions to problems that affect everyone."

In this way, what we are doing is not only about the women gathering, but it is about various groups of people gathering; young people, artists, business people, intellectuals – gathering with the intention of interrupting homogeneity. It is clear that there is a need for workable alternatives to the current status quo and we will only arrive at them through creative thinking – that is to say thinking outside of the boxes that we have been offered. It is about revival and being dynamic and seeing things with fresh eyes. Perhaps this is why I, a millennial Muslim woman in my 20s, am presenting to you today in order to bring some fresh perspectives. I was raised in a family and in a country, South Africa, where Islam is in no way traumatizing. For so many South African Muslims, it was the *deen* that brought people an inner freedom and provided a protection for them, a reminder that I am from the first generation of South Africans who did not grow up under slavery, colonialism or apartheid.

We have to remember that the conquest of Granada has a direct link with the conquest of the Americas and these methods of domination were extrapolated to the New World. It now became possible to colonise. This is a good point to introduce the first talk delivered by Aisha Bewley entitled *Colonialisation of the Deen* in which Aisha posited that today's colonialisation is the shaping of peoples' behaviors through internet and education. The age of digital capitalism has morphed into surveillance capitalism and our on-going relationship with the internet is controlling our behavior and thought processes. To quote Aisha, "all this makes old-style colonialism look amateur".

In the discussions that followed, it was clear that there was something of a split between the 'digital natives' who see the internet as a place to find community, and the 'digital immigrants' who want the amount of online activity to be as limited as possible. These two perspectives speak truth to Aisha's description of the internet as being merely a tool and not something to be feared. But the answer to the challenges presented is not something external, but instead outside, lies in a deep understanding of *tawhid* as indicated to us in Surah Kahf. Aisha concluded that the individual must find their relationship to the Divine in a profound, transformative way. Once the individual does this, he or she moves to a smaller group and from a smaller group to a larger group.

Returning to some history, this conquest of Granada and colonialisation of various parts of the world was clearly made possible through the destruction of knowledge. Thousands of books were taken from the libraries of Al-Andalus as well as from the homes of people, who had all their books confiscated, and this method was repeated in the Americas. But then, it was discovered that some knowledge was *not* contained in books at all. Knowledge of healing and health, particularly related to pregnancy and childbirth was contained within the women themselves – transmitted from generation to generation. The 'books' were in fact the bodies of these knowledgeable women, and like the Andalusian and Indigenous books, the bodies of women were burned alive. This is part of the reason for the escalation in witch hunts and persecution of women with knowledge in 15th and 16th century Europe.

Yet, while witch hunts are officially over, much of this knowledge remains compromised. In her talk *Feminine well-being in the different stages of life: The importance of the tribe*, Tahira Narbona engaged in reclaiming this knowledge, by linking wellness to *fitra*. It must also be emphasized that understanding physiology and biology is of vital importance in a world where biological differences between men and women are being obstructed and

"A true collaboration between men and women joining together to fulfill the duty of establishing a just society has not yet been realized in our lifetime."

denied even in the face of scientific evidence to the contrary.

In the discussion that followed, it was made clear that key to assisting mothers is the role of the community and the trust between women to help each other with the raising of children. The theme of this Anniversary Weekend is about the relationship between men and women, and on the subject of child rearing it was pointed out that we must create the conditions for women to be mothers and for the men to assume and take the role of the father. In order for this to happen, we must make the importance of child-rearing known to the whole community, especially the young men and the young women.

As mentioned, a vital part of motherhood is based on horizontal relationships with other women. Rahima Brandt presented on the establishment of the *awqaf* which revives other kinds of horizontal relationships and moves us away from reliance on the state. Rahima provided an overview of a *waqf* as a legal and financial instrument, covering details on how to establish one. Instead of postponing creating *awqaf* because of the magnitude of a big project such as a mosque, Rahima encouraged us to assume a genuine feminine power which is more grassroots and practical. In other words, start small. The political aspect of this cannot be ignored as these kinds of practices are anti-consumerist and re-instate the social aspect of mutual help outside the apparatus of the state.

My own talk was entitled *Resilience in a Changing Landscape* and in it, I stressed the need for women to be resilient in light of the failure to secure true liberation for women, and the need for women to be resilient in anticipation of an oncoming crisis. The danger of rhetoric was also discussed as interpreted through the following sentence from *The Time of the Bedouin,* "Rhetoric, that terrible male weapon was to silence once and for all, that unlicensed gaiety and delight and pleasure that was womanhood."

Now more than ever, there is the need for free men and free women who are not enslaved to ideology, and who are discerning and who make use of discrimination or furqan. Furthermore, I explored the need of the individual to break free of self-imposed constraints by subscribing to rhetoric and slogans on who they should be. This is not peculiar to women, but must take place for both men and women if we are to move forward.

The topics and themes we discussed during the Conference were immense and ambitious, but we also had time for music, movement, time in nature and dance. Most importantly, we made a time to do dhikr together. Rabea Redpath led a dhikr for the women and reminded us of the need to gather together for dhikr and the importance of regular recitation of the wird. In her dars, Rabea reminded us of the need for a sound heart which is the guarantee against any challenge, no matter how big or small. When faced with difficulties, we must respond with kindness and return to La ilaha illAllah. It doesn't matter if those difficulties are with the community, our families or indeed within ourselves, we respond and return to La ilaha illAllah.

Rabea also reminded us that while we have been discussing differences between men and women, at the level of the inward we are all slaves of Allah, striving to have taqwa and all on the journey to meet our Lord.

So in conclusion, I would like to say to all of the men: we need you. And you need us. And we must trust each other and we must work together. A true collaboration between men and women joining together to fulfill the duty of establishing a just society has not yet been realized in our lifetime. So it is within this intention that we find tremendous hope. Though we find ourselves in an age of civil strife and in a world whose future seems very fragile — we cannot lose hope.

I think of all those people right here in Granada in 1492, who were subject to such violence and cruelty. For them it must have appeared to be the end. How could it not? Perhaps they could not have imagined that 500 years later there would be people from all over the world coming to this city to partake in the celebration of this beautiful mosque to openly proclaim our worship of Allah and our love for the Prophet ﷺ. But perhaps among those people, were some who even in that moment of utter horror and darkness, used the light of dua. Perhaps they, with a firm intention and a high opinion of Allah, prayed for the deen to return to this place — and perhaps you all are the answer of those prayers.

IBTISAAM AHMED

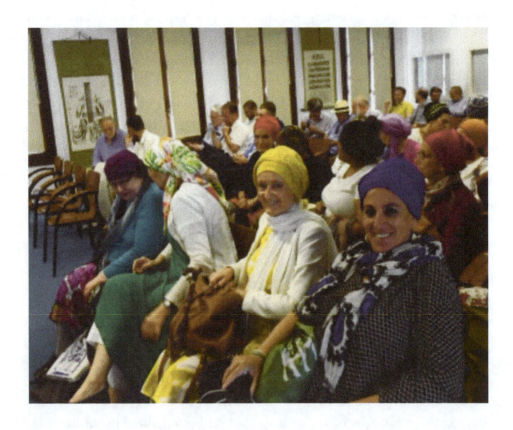

Ibtisaam Ahmed graduated with a Bachelors of Law from the University of Cape Town and a Masters of Law from Cornell University. She has taught at tertiary institutions and her research focuses on the intersection between law, history and literature. Ibtisaam is also the co-founder and managing editor of Hikaayat magazine, a platform amplifying contemporary Muslim expression.

Aisha Bewley holds a BA in French and MA in Near Eastern Languages from the University of California, Berkeley. She spent a year with a fellowship at the American University in Cairo, and was guided by Shaykh Dr. Abdalqadir as-Sufi to study with Sidi Fudul al-Huwari in Fez, Morocco. She often works with her husband Shaykh Abdalhaqq Bewley and is one of today's most prolific translators of classical Arabic texts into English including the rendering into English of the Noble Qur'an; the *Muwatta* of Imam Malik and *ash-Shifa* of Qadi Iyad. She is now working on the *Tafsir* of Qur'an by al-Qurtubi.

She is also an author in her own right, producing books such as: *Democratic Tyranny and the Islamic Paradigm*; *The Subatomic World in the Qur'an* and *Islam and the Empowering of Women*.

Rahima Brandt has a BA in Art History from UEA. She is a qualified nutritional therapist and ran a successful health supplement company until she moved to South Africa in 2005. During her time there she established a college for young Muslim women in Cape Town, which she ran until she returned to the UK. She is a passionate advocate for the revival of awqaf and is a founding member of the Local Zakat Initiative. Her other passion is printing and designing for her fabric design company. She is a mother to three girls.

Khadija Martinez was one of the main instigators and organizers of these conferences. Since she said the shahada in 1980 in Seville, she has been an active part of the Spanish and worldwide Muslim community in every way serving, by doing dawa, living and travelling throughout Europe, Turkey and South Africa, sometimes moving house and country with a few days' notice. Like the wife of the Prophet ﷺ of the same name, she has also always carried out work in the area of trading.

As she said of herself 'she graduated from the University of life.' She has started study groups of women and has always added her robust intellectual viewpoint, encouraging women to study and use their intellects.

Tahira Narbona is from Seville. She took a Diploma in Physiotherapy in 1994 having said the shahada in 1990, six months after her husband, who is a medical doctor and specialist in Family and Community medicine.

With more than twenty years of experience in the field of Physiotherapy, a diploma in Osteopathy (in 2004) and years of experience with children she is aware of the importance of female and infantile health, starting with the health of the woman herself and all the stages of development. She developed FISIOYOGA, a technique using the benefits of yoga with the therapeutic vision of physiotherapy, hormonal yoga and the recuperation of the pelvic floor. This teaching was motivated by a desire to have a holistic approach to women's health and contribute this knowledge to the community. These practices must be accompanied by a vital and natural diet and conscious exercise. She is a great advocate of natural childbirth and has accompanied various Muslim women in their home births.

Rabea Redpath has spent over forty years teaching and calling people to the deen of Islam. Since the 1970's she has been a leader and inspiration for women of all ages, with her emphasis on dhikr'Allah and the disciplines of tasawwuf. She has mentored young women in her home and gives lectures all over the world addressing the pressing issues facing Muslims in this age. Apart from her large family, the people who have lived with her and learnt from her now carry on the teaching wherever they are in England, Europe, Asia, South Africa and USA. She has always been a leading light and a source of strength for all who know her both men and women.